W9-CFW-785

The Expressiveness of the Body and the Divergence of Greek and Chinese Medicine

Shigehisa Kuriyama

ZONE BOOKS · NEW YORK

1999

© Shigehisa Kuriyama 1999

Zone Books

611 Broadway, Suite 608

New York, NY 10012

All rights reserved.

No part of this book may be reproduced, stored in
a retrieval system or transmitted in any form or by
any means, including electronic, mechanical, photo-
copying, microfilming, recording, or otherwise
(except for that copying permitted by Sections 107
and 108 of the U.S. Copyright Law and except by
reviewers for the public press) without written
permission from the Publisher.

Printed in the United States of America.

Distributed by The MIT Press,
Cambridge, Massachusetts, and London, England

Library of Congress Cataloging-in-Publication Data

Kuriyama, Shigehisa
    The expressiveness of the body and the
divergence of Greek and Chinese medicine/
Shigehisa Kuriyama.
      p. cm.
    Includes bibliographical references.
    ISBN 0-942299-88-4
1. Medicine, Chinese — Philosophy. 2. Medicine, Greek
and Roman — Philosophy. 3. Body, Human — Social
aspects. I. Title.
R723.K87 1999
610'.951 — dc21   98-37210
                                            CIP

Contents

Preface   7

PART ONE   STYLES OF TOUCHING

I   *Grasping the Language of Life*   17
II   *The Expressiveness of Words*   61

PART TWO   STYLES OF SEEING

III   *Muscularity and Identity*   111
IV   *The Expressiveness of Colors*   153

PART THREE   STYLES OF BEING

V   *Blood and Life*   195
VI   *Wind and Self*   233
Epilogue   271

Bibliographical Note   273
Notes   275
Chinese and Japanese Names and Terms   331
Index   337

Preface

Versions of the truth sometimes differ so startlingly that the very idea of truth becomes suspect. Akutagawa Ryūnosuke's haunting tale about this mystery admits two certainties: a woman has been violated by a bandit, and her husband lies in a grove, stabbed dead.

The captured bandit confesses that he killed the husband, but pleads that the woman had goaded him on. Murder hadn't been his intent — but the woman had insisted. She could not, would not tolerate two witnesses to her shame walking the earth. Kill yourself or my husband, she had said. Well, he had no choice.

Yet the woman confides that *she* killed her husband — at his own behest. As he sat silent, bound and humiliated, his eyes had spoken unmistakably of contempt and hard hatred. "Kill me," they had commanded. She realized then that they both had to die, the disgrace was too awful. But she had fainted after plunging her knife into him, and failed, finally, to end her own life.

The dead man testifies through a medium. "I killed myself," his anguished voice cries out. The horror of watching on, impotent, as his wife had first been raped and had then become enraptured, was too much. "Kill my husband," she had urged the bandit. "Take me away with you, anywhere." Death is an easy choice for a man whose wife can say such words.

7

What really happened? Was the husband murdered by his wife? By the bandit? Or was it suicide? Do even the dead deceive? Akutagawa never tells us which version to believe — or whether to believe any of them.

A similar riddle lies at the heart of the history of medicine. The true structure and workings of the human body are, we casually assume, everywhere the same, a universal reality. But then we look into history, and our sense of reality wavers. Like the confessions of the bandit, the woman, and the dead man, accounts of the body in diverse medical traditions frequently appear to describe mutually alien, almost unrelated worlds.

Compare figure 1, from Hua Shou's *Shisijing fahui* (1341) with figure 2, from Vesalius's *Fabrica* (1543). Viewed side by side, the two figures each betray lacunae. In Hua Shou, we miss the muscular detail of the Vesalian man; and in fact Chinese doctors lacked even a specific word for "muscle." Muscularity was a peculiarly Western preoccupation. On the other hand, the tracts and points of acupuncture entirely escaped the West's anatomical vision of reality. Thus, when Europeans in the seventeenth and eighteenth centuries began to study Chinese medical teachings, the descriptions of the body they encountered struck them as "phantastical" and "absurd," like tales of an imaginary land.

How can perceptions of something as basic and intimate as the body differ so? In the case of the death in the grove, we may be unsure about who is lying and who is not, and we may despair of untangling all the motives behind the liars' lies; but we have a fair idea of the forces at work. We know from our own experience how the tumult of feelings can transfigure the stories that we tell others — and ourselves. We divine in each confession chaotic mixtures of guilt and vanity, fear, anger, and self-loathing.

The parting of realities in Hua Shou and Vesalius, however,

8

presumably requires other explanations. Rather than accuse distorting passions, we are apt here to speak vaguely of different ways of thinking, or more slyly, of alternative perspectives: witnesses to an event often disagree, and not because of any dishonesty or clouded judgment, but just because of where they stand.

Yet what might "standing somewhere" involve, concretely, in the context of medical history? When we say that the first-base and home-plate umpires have different views of a play in baseball, we refer specifically to their physical locations. Each perceives aspects that the other cannot, because the two stand ninety feet apart and command different angles on the action. Clearly, such spatial positioning isn't what we mean when we speak of the disparate viewpoints of Hua Shou and Vesalius.

So what exactly *could* we mean? What sorts of distances separate "places" in the geography of medical imagination? How should we chart a map of viewpoints on the body? Such are the questions that motivate this book.

The history of medicine in China and in the West encompasses a rich variety of beliefs and practices evolving in complex patterns over several millennia. We cannot regard figures 1 and 2, therefore, or any other pair of pictures, as representing *the* Western and Chinese perspectives on the body. Neither tradition can be reduced to a single viewpoint.

Still, there is no denying the extraordinary influence — and cultural distinctiveness — of the perspectives that fixed on muscles in the one instance and acupuncture tracts in the other. It would be impossible to narrate a history of Western ideas about the structure and workings of the body without reference to muscles and muscular action; and any summary of Chinese medicine which failed to mention acupuncture tracts would be radically incomplete. Moreover, it is only over the course of the twentieth

9

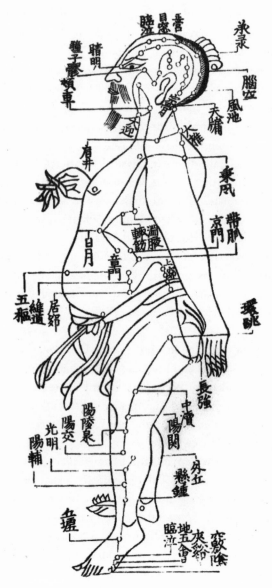

Figure 1. Hua Shou, *Shisijing fahui*, 1341, Fujikawa Collection, Kyoto University Library.

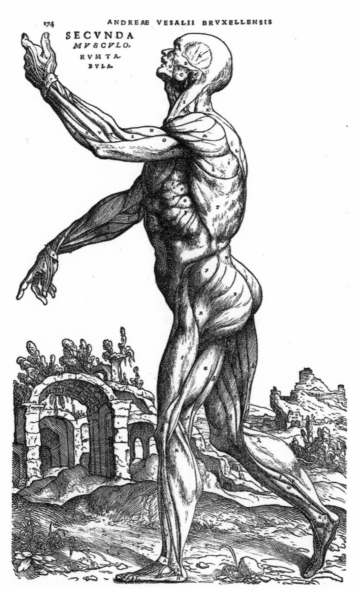

Figure 2. Veslius, *Fabrica*, 1543, Wellcome Institute, London.

Vesalius

century, with the spread of Western ideas, that muscles have become a familiar part of Chinese thinking about the body. Even now in China, complaints that English speakers express as "sore," or "tense," or "sprained muscles" are habitually experienced in other ways. By the same token, to most in the West, acupuncture, for all its recent vogue, remains a stubborn enigma. The divergence manifest in Vesalius and Hua Shou continues to inform the present.

The origins of these viewpoints long predate the two pictures. We encounter a well-developed theory of the muscular body already in the works of the Greek doctor Galen (130–200 c.e.); and by the end of the Latter Han dynasty (25–220 c.e.), which produced such canonical classics as the *Huangdi neijing* and *Nanjing*, the essential outlines of classical acupuncture would be securely in place. This is the immediate reason why the book focuses mostly on ancient medicine. For all the revisions and revolutions that subsequently transformed conceptions of the body in China and in Europe, the broad differences highlighted by figures 1 and 2 had taken shape at the latest by the turn of the second and third centuries.

On the other hand, if we delve yet deeper into the past, and examine earlier sources, such as the Hippocratic corpus and the Mawangdui manuscripts, the contrasts do not appear nearly as marked. We enter a world in which Greek doctors speak mostly of flesh and sinews rather than of muscles, and in which the Chinese art of needling has yet to be invented. This is perhaps the most compelling reason to scrutinize antiquity: such scrutiny allows us to reconsider figures 1 and 2 not as reflections of timeless attitudes, but as the results of historical change.

A major theme of the book is that conceptions of the body owe as much to particular uses of the senses as to particular "ways of

12

thinking." The distances separating figures 1 and 2 are perceptual as well as theoretical; they can never be adequately charted by intellectual schemes and sets of ideas, much less by bare formulas like holism versus dualism, organicism versus reductionism.

Part I thus details how in both Greek and Chinese medicine alike touching the body became essential to knowing the body. Chapter 1 spotlights the very distinct haptic (from the Greek *haptō*, "I touch") styles that developed in the two traditions, and chapter 2 probes the relationship between the manner in which doctors felt the expressions of the body under the fingers, and their attitudes toward the expressiveness of words.

Part II then turns to the theme of ways of seeing and examines alternative perspectives on the body as the bearer of visible meaning. Chapter 3 seeks out the specific vantage point that opened onto the vision of the muscleman, while chapter 4 explores the nature of the knowing gaze in China.

These studies of how the body was perceived from without, as an object, however, soon compel us to consider as well the problem of how the body was subjectively experienced, as it were, from within. This is the second major theme of the book: how differing ways of touching and seeing the body were bound up with different ways of *being* bodies. Part III argues that looking afresh at the history of the two substances most closely associated with vitality — namely, blood (chapter 5) and breath (chapter 6) — yields suggestive and unexpected insights into the divergence of embodied experience in China and in Europe.

The word "body," Paul Valéry observes, is commonly used to refer to a wide variety of things:

> The first is the privileged object of which, at each instant, we find ourselves in possession, although our knowledge of it — like everything that is inseparable from the instant — may be extremely vari-

13

able and subject to illusions. Each of us calls this object *My Body*; but we give it no name *in ourselves*, that is to say, *in it*. We speak of it to others as of a thing that belongs to us; but for us it is not entirely a thing; and it belongs to us a little less than we belong to it....[1]

A historical map of conceptions of the body must, this book argues, be charted in this ambiguous space between belonging and possessing, between body and self. The body is unfathomable and breeds astonishingly diverse perspectives precisely because it is a basic and intimate reality. The task of discovering the truth of the body is inseparable from the challenge of discovering the truth about people.

PART ONE

Styles of Touching

CHAPTER ONE

Grasping the Language of Life

Why hath not my soul these apprehensions, these
presages, these changes, these antidates, these jealousies, these suspicions of a sin, as well as my body of
a sickness? Why is there not always a pulse in my soul
to beat at the approach of a temptation to sin? ... I
fall sick of sin, and am bedded and bedrid, buried and
putrefied in the practice of sin, and all this while I
have no presage, no pulse, no sense of my sickness.
— John Donne, "Devotions upon Emergent
Occasions"

The truth about people is hard to know.

There is much that they will not say, and much of what they
say is only partly true. There is also much that people simply cannot say, because they themselves don't know, because many realities defy introspection. We are in the dark about the state of our
souls, John Donne laments. Turning the mind's eye inward, we
sometimes find even our bodies opaque. We may be sick without
knowing why, or in what way, or how seriously. We may be sick,
even, with no sense of sickness.

Donne hints that there is a difference, though, between bodily disorders and the diseases of the soul. Of the latter we have no inkling, no sign, our ignorance is complete. The former, by contrast, affords us "jealousies and suspicions and apprehensions of sickness before we call it a sickness" — though these are only vague premonitions, though "we are not sure we are ill." What's more, we possess a way to solve our doubts. One hand can ask "the other by the pulse ... how we do."[1] Because of the pulse, we can know the body in a way that we can never know the pulseless soul.

Once upon a time, the stirrings of the arteries commanded rapt attention. If John Donne brooded over what the pulse failed to tell him, most marveled instead at its unique revealingness. When Prince Antiochus was wasting away to the mystification of nearly all, it was again the pulse that confessed the cause. Fluttering wildly each time the prince's beautiful stepmother appeared, it whispered to a clever doctor of the torment of love, unspeakable yearning.[2] To those who could hear its message, the pulse spoke truths about a person that the person himself or herself would not or could not say.

Especially could not say. People were intensely curious about the pulse because they were intensely curious about themselves, because there were many things that they didn't know, but desperately wanted to know — such as why they felt ill, whether they would recover or die — and because they believed that the pulse could tell them.

In the second century B.C.E., in the earliest case histories of China, the sick summon Chunyu Yi not with vague pleas for succor, but with the specific wish that he come and feel their pulse. And that is just what the great doctor does. In each case, he arrives, straightaway grasps the pulse, then prescribes a remedy, explaining, "The way I knew the ailment is that when I felt the pulse...."[3] As if it were all a ritual, and his role was that of pulse interpreter.

Pulsetaking still defined the physician nearly two millennia later, when the novelist Cao Xueqin (d. 1763) portrayed the tangle of hopes and subtle suspicions that made this act so thick with meaning.

"Is this the lady?" asked the doctor.

"Yes, this is my wife," Jia Rong replied. "Do sit down! I expect you would like me to describe her symptoms first, before you feel her pulse?"

"If you permit me, no," said the doctor. "I think it would be better if I felt the pulse first and asked you about the development of the illness afterwards. This is the first time I have been to your house, and as I am not a skilled practitioner and have only come here at our friend Mr. Feng's insistence, I think I should feel the pulse and give you my diagnosis first. We can go on to talk about her symptoms and discuss a course of treatment if you are satisfied with the diagnosis. And of course, it will still be up to you to decide whether or not the treatment I prescribe is to be followed."

"You speak with real authority, doctor," said Jia Rong. "I only wish we had got to hear of you earlier. Feel her pulse, then, and let us know whether she can be cured, so that my parents may be spared further anxiety."[4]

For over two thousand years, in China, in Europe, and elsewhere too, people queried the pulse with passionate interest. In principle, Chinese doctors recognized four ways to judge a person's condition — gazing (*wang*), listening and smelling (*wen*), questioning (*wen*), and touching (*qie*). In practice, however, their attentions concentrated mainly on *qiemo*, palpating the *mo*. Look at what they wrote: no monographs devoted to diagnostic listening or smelling; no essays on techniques of interrogation; over 150 works on the interpretation of haptic signs.[5]

We find a similar enthusiasm in Western medicine. In antiquity, the Greek physician Galen composed seven extended treatises on the pulse, filling nearly a thousand pages of his collected works. In the sixteenth century, Hercules Saxonia declared that "Nothing is or ever will be more significant in medical science."[6] Benjamin Rush reasoned for his part that if admission into Plato's Temple of Philosophy required mastery of geometry, the gates to a Temple of Medicine should bear the inscription "Let no one enter here who is not acquainted with the pulse."[7] Even in 1878, an American doctor could still pronounce pulsetaking "the most valuable of all the devices to which a physician can resort," and think himself echoing "the unanimous voice" of his colleagues.[8]

Things are different in modern medicine, of course. Past interpretations of the pulse's murmurings have largely been exiled to the netherworld of antiquarian lore. So it is worth remembering: *some* telling connection binds pulsing and life. No one can doubt this.

A person with a beating pulse still lives. Someone whose pulse has stopped is dead. And we can check for ourselves, at our own wrists, that the pulse changes noticeably, and in distinctive ways, when we eat breakfast, or chase after a departing bus, or stand shivering in the rain. The question of how pulsing relates to life concerns not just the beliefs of people in distant eras and lands, but the logic governing our own lives, here and now.

In how many ways, and why, can, and does the pulse change? Julius Rucco once characterized the pulse as nature's means of speaking to the doctor — the language of life.[9] But what then is its grammar, its vocabulary? Doctors said that they knew. For two millennia, much of their authority to mediate between patients and their own bodies turned on their supposed mastery of this secret idiom.

Yet the languages mastered by Chinese and European physicians were not at all the same.

Seventeenth-century travelers to China marveled at the astonishing prowess of local healers, and especially at their exquisite feel for the pulse. The uncanny accuracy of their diagnoses bordered on the incredible. Chinese doctors, Thomas Baker concluded cautiously from missionary reports, apparently had "such skill in pulses, as is not to be imagined but by those that are acquainted with them."[10] "All the accounts of travelers," remarks Diderot's *Encyclopédie*, "agree in presenting the doctors of this country as wonderful (*merveilleux*) in this art."[11] Cures like acupuncture and moxibustion were intriguing, too; but up through the nineteenth century, talk of medicine in China first called to mind this "skill in pulses."

From the very outset, however, this art posed a conundrum. When Michael Boym's (1612–59) Latin translation of the *Mojue* (a popular Chinese pulse manual) began to circulate in Europe, it left readers utterly baffled. "The missionary who sent this account," commented William Wotton, "was afraid that it would be thought ridiculous by Europeans; which fear of his seems to have been well-grounded."[12] Chinese tenets struck him as not just mistaken but absurd. They literally made no sense. The author of the *Encyclopédie* article, too, judged the exposé of Chinese doctrines "an impenetrable chaos."[13] Even John Floyer, perhaps the most enthusiastic early champion of Chinese medicine, had to concede that its teachings about the pulse were sometimes "very obscure" and "phantastical."

Floyer urged, nonetheless, that the "absurd notions" of the Chinese were "adjusted to the real phenomena";[14] and he set out to "prove . . . that the Chinese have found out the real art of feeling the pulse." After all, they got results.[15] Floyer's formula sum-

21

marizes the tension that long defined European assessments of palpation in China. In his authoritative text on the physiology of the pulse (1886), Charles Ozanam ridiculed Chinese pulse theory, scoffing that in them "the allegorical triumphs over the real." But he also added: "One would be tempted to abandon its study were it not for the fact that the most reliable witnesses assure us that by their science of the pulse, the Chinese recognize and cure, sometimes with extraordinary success, the most recalcitrant illnesses."[16]

Here then was a technique that looked so familiar, and allegedly worked wonders in practice, but whose discourse seemed completely alien and misguided. Travelers watched native doctors place their fingers on patients' wrists and immediately recognized the gesture of feeling the pulse. By the evidence of the eyes, *qiemo*, palpating the *mo*, was unmistakably pulse diagnosis.

Chinese writings testified that the eyes were wrong. The hermeneutics of the *Mojue* were unlike any dialect of the pulse language known in Europe.[17]

How can gestures look the same, yet differ entirely in the experience? When three blind men were queried about the nature of the elephant, one replied that it resembled a long, thin rope, another that it was like a stubby, thick pillar, and the third that it was an immense sack. The three disagreed because the first had grasped the elephant's tail, the second had embraced a leg, and the third was running his hands over the stomach. But they didn't know this. Each knew only that he was right, and each was bewildered by the delusions of the others. All three had real knowledge of the same elephant. Yet what each knew was absolutely different.

Much the same could be said about European doctors feeling the pulse and Chinese doctors feeling the *mo*. Despite the similarities in appearance, and despite the fact the two procedures ostensibly examined the "same" place, pulse diagnosis and *qiemo* entailed perceptions as disparate as grabbing the elephant's tail and rubbing its stomach. I spoke above of Chinese doctors taking the "pulse"; English affords no better approximation. But it is only an approximation, and charting its limits compels us to re-think much of what we take for granted in the body.

Like the pulse. The very idea.

The Birth of the Pulse

Our knowledge of classical Greek medicine derives chiefly from two sources. The first is the collection of treatises composed mostly between 450 and 350 B.C.E. and attributed to Hippocrates of Cos; the second are the voluminous works of Galen (129–200 C.E.).[18] The latter includes extensive, detailed discussions of the pulse, elaborating its causes and functions, its varieties and use in prognosis. Remarkably, however, half a millennium earlier, in the Hippocratic corpus, we hear nothing of pulsetaking. Indeed, Hippocratic physicians seem scarcely even to have recognized a concept of "pulse." Interrogating the pulse is not some inevitable, prehistoric instinct.

How did the practice come into being? The pulse has been so basic for so long to the Western understanding of the body that we tend, thoughtlessly, to suppose it beyond history. We ask, "How did Chinese physicians interpret the pulse?" as if "the pulse" were a natural given, a fixed, universal reality perceived differently by different peoples — something perhaps like Jastrow's rabbit duck (figure 3), in which one person sees a rabbit and another a duck. Yes, the pulse was "overlooked" by Hippocratic physicians, those keen observers. But our impulse is to regard this as a perceptual lapse, an odd failure to notice something already there, waiting to be noticed.

This is where comparisons are enlightening.

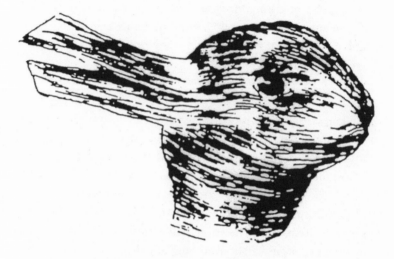

Figure 3. Jastrow's rabbit/duck from Norma V. Scheidemann, *Experiments in General Psychology* (Chicago: University of Chicago Press, 1939).

What do we feel when we place our fingers on the wrist, and palpate the movements there? We say: the pulsing artery. What else could there be? Chinese doctors performing the same gesture, however, grasped a more complex reality (figure 4). The finger placed lightly on the right wrist, at the *cun* position, diagnosed the large intestines, while the finger next to it discerned the state of the stomach. Pressing harder, these two fingers probed, respectively, the flourishing or decline of the lungs and spleen. Under each finger, then, doctors separated a superficial (*fu*) site, felt near the body surface, from a sunken (*chen*) site deeper down. There were thus six pulses under the index, middle, and ring fingers, and twelve pulses on the two wrists combined.

Small wonder that Floyer and Wotton were perplexed. To describe twelve pulses at the wrist is to describe something other than the pulse. But if not the pulse, then what? No sooner do we ask this than we are led to question the reality hitherto taken for granted: What *is* the pulse, and how did it come to be?

The *Synopsis on Pulses*, attributed to Rufus of Ephesus, opens with an intriguing clue about the beginnings of Greek pulse study: "It is necessary to study the art of the pulse carefully, for without it it is impossible to design suitable treatment. It is said that Aegimius, the first who wrote on this matter, took for title not *On Pulses* (*Peri sphygmōn*), but rather *On Palpitations* (*Peri palmōn*), for he did not know, it seems, that there is a difference between pulse and palpitation, as we will show in what follows."[19] Rufus thus names the first writer on sphygmology. Unfortunately, the name is all we have, and we know virtually nothing about Aegimius.[20] The title of Aegimius' treatise, on the other hand, is rather suggestive.

It poses a puzzle. Why should a work on the pulse be called *On Palpitations*? Galen also found the title odd, and faulted Aegi-

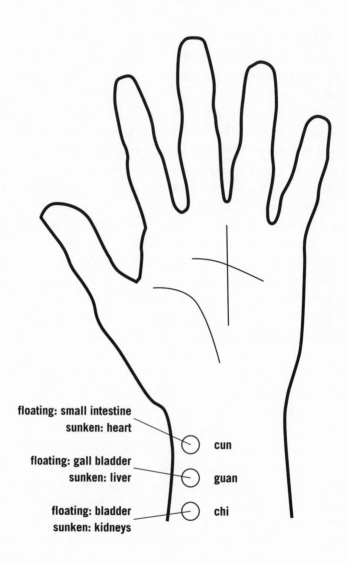

floating: small intestine
sunken: heart
cun

floating: gall bladder
sunken: liver
guan

floating: bladder
sunken: kidneys
chi

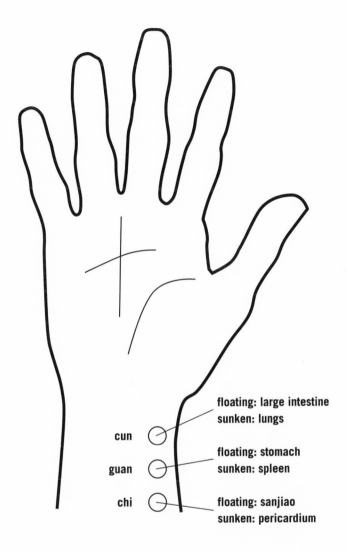

cun floating: large intestine
sunken: lungs

guan floating: stomach
sunken: spleen

chi floating: sanjiao
sunken: pericardium

Figure 4. Qiemo sites.

mius' unconventionality. Contrary to both standard medical usage and to common parlance, Aegimius called "palpitation" what Praxagoras and Herophilus would later, more properly, call "pulse."[21] Rufus, for his part, blamed a subtler ignorance. Aegimius just wasn't yet aware of the distinction between pulse and palpitation. His title reflected the confusions of an earlier, more primitive understanding of the body. In any event, *On Palpitations* struck both Rufus and Galen as a misleading title. Already by their time, that is, by the time of the earliest *extant* writings on the pulse, the meanings of key terms had changed.

Aegimius actually wasn't alone in his "confusion." In Hippocratic writings as well, *sphygmos*, Rufus' and Galen's term for the pulse, formed a continuum with *palmos* (palpitation), *tromos* (tremor), and *spasmos* (spasm). It named a minor pathological sign of only occasional note. References to it are scarce.[22] The verb *sphyzein* referred not to the constant physiological activity of the arteries, not to what we call "pulsing," but rather to the throbbing that sometimes accompanies fevers and inflammations.[23] Thus, *Fractures* speaks of a "throbbing and inflamed" injury, and *Wounds* describes how "a wound becomes inflamed, and then shivering and throbbing ensue."[24] More remarkably still, *Epidemics* 2 cites as a telling sign the fact that both hands of the patient "pulsed" — as if even pulsing at the wrist was a pathological aberration.[25] At the start, then, sphygmos did not evoke a pulse that beats day in and day out from birth to death.[26] The Hippocratic body had no natural beat.[27]

On reflection, this may not be so strange. In daily life, most of us rarely if ever attend to the pulse. Pulsation intrudes into our consciousness only in extraordinary states, like the throbbing of pain or duress. It is just historical habit — the long tradition of pulse taking — that makes interest in pulsation seem self-evident and instinctive.

Two philological details hint at the chasm separating pre- from post-sphygmological consciousness. First, there is the term *sphygmoi*, or "pulses." Several Hippocratic passages deploy this plural where we expect the singular. *Diseases of Women* speaks of "the pulses quivering, faint, and fading against the hand"; *Epidemics* 4 relates that, "the pulses of Zoilos the carpenter were trembling and obscure."[28] Note well: it wasn't the carpenter's *pulse* that trembled and was obscure, but his pulse*s*. *Sphygmoi* named throbbings and pulsing in their concrete multiplicity; the idea of *the* pulse had yet to crystallize. In later Greek medicine, by contrast, the plural *sphygmoi* would designate the plurality of pulse types. Galen's title, *On Differences between Pulses (Peri diaphorās sphygmōn)*, refers to the variety of pulses, such as the large pulse, the small pulse, the quick pulse, and the slow pulse. In diagnosing a specific person at a specific time, Galen always speaks of the patient's pulse, not pulses.

The second characteristic of Hippocratic usage is the close association of *sphygmos* and *palmos*, of pulse and palpitation. To Hippocrates' contemporaries, Aegimius' title *On Palpitations* probably wouldn't have seemed peculiar. Hippocratic treatises frequently paired pulse and palpitation, and used them in ways that are hard to distinguish. Blood vessels (*phlebes*) "palpitate" as often as they "pulse," and often they do both.[29] Nor was *sphygmos* confined to the blood vessels. It appeared equally in the head, in the hypochondrium, in the womb.[30]

Palmos and *sphygmos*, in short, both named abnormal movements in the blood vessels and elsewhere, and the difference between them was frequently unclear.[31] We have late testimony, however, for the views of Praxagoras of Cos, a renowned physician not far removed from the time of Hippocrates.[32] According to Rufus and Galen, Praxagoras believed that palpitation was only pulsing of great intensity. He maintained, further, that trembling (*tromos*) was in turn just a violent palpitation, and spasm (*spasmos*) just intensified trembling.[33] Pulsations, palpitations, tremors, and spasms thus formed a continuum.

There would eventually be a divinatory art devoted to these motions. Palmomantics, one of the superstitions attacked by Christian authors such as Augustine, assigned prophetic meaning to the sudden jerks, twitchings, and throbbings of the body. Beating in the right temple portended greatness and power, and the abuse of slaves; in the right eyebrow, it foretold a short sickness; between the eyebrows, misfortune for all — except for the slave, for whom it meant good luck; in the upper eyelid of the right eye, health and success. This was a minor art; only one treatise, Melampus's *On Palpitations*, survives.[34] By Melampus' time, another, more promising system of somatic interpretation had already arisen — sphygmology, a science that segregated a single kind of motion from all the others.

How do pulse and palpitation differ? Galen reports that Herophilus, the founder of Greek sphygmology, began his book on the pulse with precisely this question. Rufus' *Synopsis on Pulses*, too, after its opening definition of the pulse, jumps straight to the differences that distinguish it from palpitations, spasms, and tremors.[35] For early Greek expositors of the pulse, the divorce of *sphygmos* from *palmos* represented the first and decisive step toward defining this new realm of study.

Basic to this divorce was the new perception of the body defined by dissection. Anatomy helped to transform *sphygmos* from a vague occasional oddity into a vital sign. The earliest extensive evidence of systematic anatomy appears in the animal dissections of Aristotle; and it is also in Aristotle that we first catch glimmerings of *sphygmos* as a regular physiological phenomenon. In his treatise *On Respiration*, Aristotle notes that "All the vessels throb (*sphyzousin*), and throb simultaneously with each other, because

30

they are connected with the heart,"[36] and he even distinguishes the heart's pulsation from its palpitation.[37] To be sure, he makes no mention of the medical use of the pulse; indeed, he still had yet to separate arteries from veins. His *sphygmos* was still not the pulse of Herophilus and Galen. But his inquiries already adumbrate the ties binding the birth of the pulse idea to the inspection of dissected structures.

Anatomy framed the very possibility of imagining the pulse. Take Rufus' formula: "The pulse is the diastole and systole of the heart and the arteries"[38] — to us a seemingly self-evident definition, yet one for which Hippocratic doctors had not even the words. The artery/vein dichotomy was alien to the system of "veins" (*phlebes*) traced in treatises like *On the Sacred Disease* and *On the Nature of the Human Being.*[39] *Phlebes*, moreover, stretched the length of the body in routes that cannot be directly matched with anatomical blood vessels. Indeed, in these treatises they don't even all spring from, nor return to, the heart. Suggestively, the individual hailed as the founder of pulse study is also the physician credited with pioneering human dissection. I speak of Herophilus.[40]

It is instructive to compare Herophilus' views with those of his teacher Praxagoras. Apparently, Praxagoras also took an interest in both dissection and pulsation, and may even have taken the first steps toward distinguishing arteries from veins.[41] But he reportedly conceived of nerves as the refined extensions of the arterioles. Nerves and arteries, he thought, both carried pneuma and served as the conduits by which the heart controlled the movement of muscles.[42] This scheme possibly underlay his view of the continuity between *sphygmos*, *palmos*, *tromos*, and *spasmos* — his belief that pulse and palpitation differed only in intensity, not in kind. Thus "*sphygmos* turns into *palmos* as its motion grows faster, and from *palmos* arises *tromos*."[43]

31

Herophilus thus set out, Galen informs us, "at the very start of his book about pulses to refute this doctrine of his teacher."[44] And therein lies his claim to found sphygmology. It was Herophilus who determined that "the pulse exists only in the arteries and heart, whereas palpitation, spasm, and tremor appear in the muscles and nerves."[45] It was he, not Praxagoras, who demonstrated that arteries and nerves were distinct, and that the pulse belonged uniquely to the former. Once pulse, palpitation, spasm, and tremor were parsed according to their subtending structures, their haptic similarities could no longer confuse. The pulse was no more a type of spasm than arteries were a sort of nerve.

By separating blood vessels from nerves, and among blood vessels, arteries from veins, anatomy thus helped forge the object of sphygmological study. But that isn't all. It also, and more subtly, framed the method of study. This point can scarcely be overemphasized. Anatomy shaped how and what the fingers felt.

How do the heart and arteries known to the eye relate to the experience of the fingers? Greek sphygmology was born with the assertion that whatever similarities they might present to the touch, pulsation, palpitation, tremor, and spasm differ in the structures that underlie them. Palpitations, tremblings, and spasms all belong to the nervelike parts of the body, Herophilus discovered. The pulse, on the other hand, occurs only in the arteries and the heart. Further, the pulse "is born with a living being and dies with it, whereas these other motions do not. Also the pulse ... occurs both when the arteries are filled and when they are emptied, whereas these others do not; and the pulse at all times attends us involuntarily and exists naturally, whereas the others are within our power to choose...."[46]

Bacchius similarly defined the pulse as "the diastole and systole occurring simultaneously in all the arteries";[47] for Heraclides of Erythrae it was "the dilation and systole of the arteries accomplished by the prevailing natural and psychic power";[48] and Aristoxenus would characterize it more specifically as "an activity of the heart and arteries that is peculiar to them."[49] From the start, the idea of the pulse was inseparable from the image of the pulsing artery.

Inseparable, but of course not identical: the artery was a visible structure, the pulse was a set of motions. Moreover, these motions were largely inaccessible to sight; the pulse had to be *felt*. From this situation sprang the most vexed problem in pulse study, namely, that of how the arteries seen in dissection were linked to what the fingers now sensed.

What *do* we mean by the pulse? Most ancient definitions, like those of Hēgētōr, Bacchius, and Heraclides, required imagining motions in the mind's eye: they spoke of arteries dilating and contracting, of diastole and systole. This represented the mainstream. Though accounts of the cause and function of pulsation changed considerably in the two thousand years after Herophilus, picturing the tubular artery remained throughout the enduring basis of Western pulse analysis.

Yet some in antiquity already expressed qualms. In particular, physicians of the empiricist school insisted on the distance separating the anatomical definition of the pulse and the actual experience of the fingers. What our fingers feel, the empiricists contended, is merely the sensation of being struck. We don't actually perceive the artery expanding and contracting. We only *infer* diastole and systole.[50] Empirically, the pulse is nothing more than a series of beats and pauses.

Nor were the empiricists alone in suggesting limits to haptic knowledge. Herophilus' follower Alexander, for instance, promoted a two-part definition: in terms of its essential nature, objectively, the pulse was "the involuntary systole and diastole of

33

the heart and arteries"; but to actual inspection (*episkepsei*), sub-jectively, it was merely "the striking against the touch produced by the completely involuntary motion of the arteries, and the rest the interval that follows the striking."[51] Alexander's disciple Demos-thenes advanced the same two-tiered scheme in his three treatises on the pulse, and these works reportedly commanded respect.[52]

Such debates help to explain the convolutions in Galen's version:

> We detect in several parts of the skin some sort of motion, and this not only by pressing down on them, but sometimes with our eyes as well. Moreover this motion is found among all healthy people in many parts of the body — of which one is the wrist. [In such places] we can clearly detect something coming from below up to the skin and striking against us; after the beat, sometimes it distinctly moves away and then pauses, and sometimes right after the beginning [of motion] it appears to pause, and then comes again and beats, and then it goes away again and rests. And this process goes on in the entire body, from the day we are born until we die. It is this type of motion that all people call the pulse.[53]

Plainly displayed in this account are the molding pressures of empiricist doubt. No mention here even of arteries, much less of their diastole or systole. Galen starts instead by affirming the occasional visibility of pulsation. The pulse, he implies, is not inferred but directly perceived. Insisting, he asserts elsewhere that in thin individuals with large pulses even the artery's con-traction can be observed by the naked eye.[54]

Visual evidence forms just part of Galen's defense, however. His main argument is that diastole and systole are tactile truths. We can really feel, he declares, much more than the bare beats and pauses recognized by the empiricists. Our fingers can directly follow the artery as it moves toward and away from them; indeed, they can catch even the pauses punctuating these opposing movements. In affirming anatomical knowledge, we needn't slight the experience of the touch: ultimately, the two converge.

Is this true? Can the artery's systole really be felt? Opinions differed. Herophilus included the systole as part of the pulse, and this, combined with his stress on basing knowledge on experience, suggested to many that he had known it as an empirical fact. Certainly most of his followers conceived the systole in this way. Others weren't so sure. Archigenes affirmed that the contraction could be felt, while Agathinus held that it couldn't.[55] The pneumatically inspired *Medical Definitions* opposed the direct experience of the diastole to the inferred character of the systole.[56]

Galen decided that he had to judge for himself. For a long time, despite striving strenuously to refine his touch, he found it impossible to follow the artery in its contractions. More than once, he thought of giving up. Then, suddenly one day, a flash of enlightenment.[57] He grasped it: the systole was knowable by the touch after all. Though he confessed: "Final knowledge seems to require all of a lifetime."[58]

Try, yourself, to perceive more than beats and pauses, to follow the swell and fall of the artery, and you appreciate Galen's toils. Did you really feel the contraction? Or just imagine it? How can you be sure? The motion is so quick. You probably would never feel it if you didn't anticipate it. But does the anticipation then corrupt the experience?

There is something dreamlike about the history of generations upon generations of physicians struggling in this way, each concentrating furiously for months, years, on tiny motions of eye-blink swiftness flickering under their fingers, each trying desperately to sort out genuine perceptions from inferences and

35

hallucinations. Many believed, however, that there was no other way truly to understand the pulse. According to Herophilus, the pulse communicated its message through these elements: size, speed, strength, rhythm, order and disorder, regularity and irregularity. Except for strength, all these required taking the exact measure, in space and in time, of the expanding and receding artery.

In Galen's analysis, size was composed of length, breadth, and height. Along each dimension, the artery's dilation might be excessive (long, broad, high), deficient (short, narrow, or low), or in between. Speed pitted the distance the arterial wall moved against the time consumed in the motion. Gauging this meant splitting fleeting moments into the thinnest instants. For Galen taught that a single pulse comprised four parts: the diastole, the rest following diastole and preceding systole, the systole, and the rest following systole and preceding diastole.[59] One thus had to separate the durations of the motions from the durations of the rests.

Frequency hinged on the duration of the rests. The shorter the rests, the more frequent the pulse. Since Galen posited two rests, he identified two frequencies: one determined by the "outer rest" (between the end of diastole and the start of systole), the other fixed by the "inner rest" (between the end of systole and the start of diastole). Rhythm was the ratio of the durations of the systole and the diastole. Unevenness and irregularity measured the relative durations of diastole, systole, and also the two rests.

Seizing the pulse thus entailed seizing changes more easily imagined than grasped. We can readily picture the walls of a dilating and contracting tube, and dissect its size, speed, frequency, and rhythm, neatly and geometrically in the mind's eye.[60] Discerning all these by the touch is much harder. Yet that was the task.

Someone who attended only to beats and pauses would miss

36

the bulk of the pulse's confidences, would catch merely muffled rumblings. The language of the pulse was an idiom of diastole and systole. Beyond rooting the pulse in the heart and the arteries, anatomy defined what and how doctors trained their fingers to feel.

Today it is nearly impossible to shake the hold of this tradition. You put your fingers on the wrists and you immediately envision the pulsing artery, as a matter of course. You can scarcely even imagine what else you could feel. And yet no necessity dictates the pulsetaker's approach. There are other ways to cradle meaning at the wrist. As palpation in China makes plain.

Qiemo

Against skeptics who rejected Chinese pulse teachings because of their "mistakes in anatomy," John Floyer argued in 1707 "that the want of anatomy does make their art very obscure, and gives occasion to use phantastical notions; but their absurd notions are adjusted to the real phenomena, and their art is grounded upon curious experience, examined and approved for four thousand years."[61]

By the early nineteenth century, however, most European doctors seemed to agree with the stance of Johan L. Formey when, in his *Versuch einer Wurdigung des Pulses* (1823), he airily dismissed Chinese pulse theory as idle sophistry. It couldn't be otherwise since any theory of the pulse that floated free of a "fundamental anatomical knowledge of the human body" had to remain error-ridden.[62]

At the start of the twentieth century, the Chinese physician Tang Zonghai noted the same conflict between *qiemo* tenets and the findings of dissection, but drew the opposite conclusion. The efficacy of traditional palpation, he contended, exposed the limitations of anatomy: "Western physicians don't believe in the

37

method of the *mo*. They say that the *mo* which circulate around the body all arise from the blood vessels of the heart, that it is because of the ceaseless activity of the heart that the *mo* move. But how can the condition of the five viscera be determined by just the blood vessels? They further talk of the *mo* of the hand being a single pathway. But then how could it be divided into *cun*, *guan*, and *chi*?"[63]

Experience showed that by palpating the *mo* doctors could diagnose not just the heart, but all the viscera; showed, too, that the wrist comprised several sites, not just one. That dissection suggested otherwise proved only that dissection could mislead. Qian Depei argued likewise that, although Western medicine excelled in anatomy, Chinese medicine excelled in palpation. The future of medicine lay in their combination.[64] In any event, Tang and Qian concurred with Western doctors on one point: Chinese palpation wasn't based on the imagination of the dilating and contracting artery. The *mo* wasn't the pulse.

Travelers who wrote back to Europe with the first reports of Chinese palpation saw a technique that looked identical to pulse taking. Doctors silently felt the wrist for a long time and then announced what was wrong. However, if we consult the *Huangdi neijing* or simply *Neijing*, the oldest and most revered of the Chinese medical classics, we find a rather greater variety of techniques.[65] In the *Suwen* and the *Lingshu*, the two texts that compose the *Neijing*, palpation concentrated on the wrist alone appears as merely one technique among several, and not even the most popular one at that. At the start, other strategies held more sway.[66]

The *Lingshu* especially promoted comparison of the *mo* at the wrist with that at the neck. The latter revealed the body's yang powers, the former, the yin powers. A *mo* at the neck twice stronger

38

than that at the wrist, for instance, indicated a "Greater Yang" condition — an ailment in the bladder and small intestines. Conversely, a *mo* twice stronger at the wrist meant a "Greater Yin" affliction, affecting the spleen or lungs.[67]

Treatise 20 of the *Suwen* favored comparing nine sites (eighteen total, adding together the sites on the right and left sides): three on the head, three on the arm, and three on the feet. Each gave insight into a separate part of the body. The movements at the temple, for example, announced the condition of the eyes and ears, the movements at the wrist corresponded to the lungs, and the movements behind the ankle to the kidneys.[68]

Suwen treatise 17 outlined a third technique, which postulated twelve sites at the *cunkou*, or "inch-opening" at the wrists.[69]

	Left wrist	Right wrist
Upper (*shang*)		
Outer (*wai*)	Heart	Lungs
Inner(*nei*)	*danzhong*	Thorax
Middle (*zhong*)		
Outer	Liver	Stomach
Inner	Diaphragm	Spleen
Lower (*xia*)		
Outer	Kidneys	Kidneys
Inner	Abdomen	Abdomen

The disposition of sites thus roughly mirrored the spatial organization of the body. The upper position corresponded to the body above the diaphragm, the middle position to between the diaphragm and the navel, and the lower position to the lower body.[70]

The *Nanjing*, the classic exploring "difficulties" (*nan*) raised by the *Neijing*, subsequently replaced plain everyday words like "upper," "middle," and "lower," "outer" and "inner," with the technical vocabulary of *cun*, *guan*, and *chi*, "floating" (*fu*) and "sunken" (*chen*). Wang Shuhe's *Mojing*, the canonical compilation on the *mo*, further eliminated the repetitions in the *Suwen* scheme and matched inspection sites with specific yin and yang viscera rather than with broad areas such as the abdomen and the thorax (figure 4).

Even the *Mojing* wasn't the final word. When the eighteenth-century Japanese doctor Katō Munehiro reviewed the evolution of Chinese palpation, he counted no less than eight distinct ways to feel the wrist, each matching sites with viscera in disparate ways.[71] *Qiemo* thus wasn't a single, timeless system, but encompassed a congery of approaches that continued to be revised.

A unifying assumption, however, ran through them all. All approaches took for granted that the meaning of *what* the fingers felt, depended on *where* they felt. When it appeared under the index finger, a given quality might signal recovery, under the middle finger, continued decline. As one doctor summed up: "Although the three fingers are separated by mere hairbreadths, the diseases they indicate are a thousand leagues apart."[72] Chinese debates about palpation almost all revolved around the issues of which sites the diagnostician should examine, and what each implied. If the *mo* was the language of life, its grammar was topological.

Comparatively viewed, this is perhaps the most salient characteristic of palpation in China: the belief in the significance of place. From Herophilus through Galen, Greek diagnosticians evinced little interest in, or even awareness of, the differing feel of the pulse in distant parts. Galen merely remarks that one inspects the wrist because the pulse there can be felt clearly and without offending the patient's modesty.[73] The idea of systematically comparing alternative sites never arises.[74] Why should it? Since the arteries all spring from the heart, doctors expected traits like speed, frequency, and rhythm to be the same in them all.

But those traits do not exhaust what can be felt, and other qualities do not always manifest themselves uniformly everywhere. Again, check yourself. Monitor the pulses in your left and right wrists and you may find that on a given day the left pulse feels harder or bigger than the right, yet on another day the reverse may be true. Chinese doctors deliberately sought out such variations and shifts. *Qiemo* was not a science of the pulse.

What was palpation of the *mo* all about? A wise minister in the *Zuozhuan* warns the marquis of Jin that foreign-bred horses, unaccustomed to the local climate and people, will fluster easily; and he conjures up the image of their frantic panting, blood pounding through their bodies, their *mo* bulging taut, standing out. We picture the veins of the nervous steeds, made tumescent by fear, excitement, and the rush of blood. This is the earliest reference to the *mo*.[75] Originally, *mo* evoked blood vessels.

Until a few decades ago, historical analysis of the *mo* in medicine would have had to begin with the *Neijing*. But in 1973, some remarkable manuscripts were unearthed from the Mawangdui tombs at Changsha. Composed or copied probably sometime between the third century B.C.E. and 168 B.C.E. (the date of the tombs) — that is, before the compilation of the *Neijing* — they have forced historians to rethink the development of classical Chinese medicine. Two texts in particular shed fresh light on the evolution of ancient thinking about the *mo*. Modern scholars have dubbed them the *Zubi shiyimo jiujing* (Treatise on the moxibustion of the eleven *mo* of the legs and arms) and the *Yinyang shiyimo jiujing* (Treatise on the moxibustion of the eleven yin and yang *mo*).[76]

41

Portions of major arteries and veins can be recognized in portions of each of the *mo* described in these texts, especially as they become visible near the joints — the neck, ankles, knees, elbows, wrists. Recurrent references to the *mo* "emerging" and "entering" at these junctures reveal how blood vessels visible at the body surface remained, as in the *Zuozhuan* tale of frightened horses, integral to the imagination of the *mo*.

But none of the *mo* corresponds directly to particular arteries or veins. The Greater Yang Leg Mo, for example, emerges from the outer ankle, rises up through the back of the lower leg, and emerges at the knee. At this point it splits in two, with one branch servicing the thigh, and another running up along the spine and into the back of the head. There it splits again, with one branch terminating in the ear, and another running through the eye into the nose.[77] No major blood vessel matches these meanderings from ankle to eye.

Even more telling is the silence about the heart. The Mawangdui *mo* neither arise from nor return to the heart, and no interconnections seem to bind them together. They run between the head and trunk and the legs and arms like eleven independent tracts. The *mo* were not the arteries or veins of the anatomist. Only partly did their explanation lie in blood vessels seen from the outside. More decisive was the inner experience of pain.

Uniting the disparate places through which the *mo* coursed was the thread of affliction and its relief. Aching twinges in the lower leg, spasms of the knee, agony gripping the lower back and buttocks, hearing difficulties, and prickly pain around the eyes — all found relief in the same cure: burning moxa on the Greater Yang Mo. And so it went for all the conduits. The Teeth Mo, the Eye Mo, and the Shoulder Mo owed their names mainly to the fact that cauterizing these *mo* relieved discomfort, respectively, in the teeth, the eyes, and the shoulders. Crucial to conceiving what

42

the *mo* were and where they wandered were observations about how and why treating one site on the body solved suffering in other, distant parts.

The connections drawn by the *Zubi shiyimo* and *Yinyang shiyimo* show them unmistakably to be the near ancestors of the conduits, the *jing* or *jingmo*, of acupuncture. The pathology and trajectory of the Greater Yang Leg Mo in the *Zubi shiyimo* closely approximate those of the Greater Yang Bladder vessel later needled in the *Neijing*; and we can similarly identify the acupuncture correlates of the ten other *mo* as well. The Mawangdui manuscripts, in short, offer a window onto the origins of the acupuncture body portrayed in figure 1.

What was the genealogy of conduit theory in ancient China? Ma Jixing and others have compared the Mawandui treatises with each other and with *Lingshu* treatise 10 and studied the theoretical elaboration of the *mo* from the end of the Warring States period (476–221 B.C.E.) through the Qin (221–206 B.C.E.) and Western Han (206 B.C.E.– 8 C.E.) dynasties.[78] The process almost certainly involved multiple lines of development: a lacquer conduit-figurine recovered from a Western Han tomb in 1993 depicts only nine *mo*, even though it ostensibly dates from after the Mawangdui treatises describing eleven *mo*. Moreover, two of the *mo* etched on the figurine are ones that these treatises don't discuss.[79]

But the most startling feature of the pre-*Neijing* evidence (including the lacquer figurine) is the absence of any reference to acupuncture points, or, for that matter, to acupuncture. Both the *Zubi shiyimo* and the *Yinyang shiyimo* speak only of treating particular *mo*, without specifying particular sites; furthermore, the treatment they prescribe is moxibustion, not needling.

Lu Shouyan speculated in the 1950s that primitive healers began by discovering the efficacy of needling particular points, then gradually inferred a series of channels to link them together; and this was long thought a plausible story.[80] However, the discovery of the Mawangdui texts has raised serious doubts, and Yamada Keiji, for one, has recently advanced the opposite scenario, urging that the discovery of the *mo* preceded the discovery of points.[81] At the very least, it now seems possible, perhaps even probable, that theories of the *mo* developed independently of a theory of points.

Yet if the *mo* weren't inferred from points, how did belief in them originally arise? Current evidence supports no definite view on the matter — though I shall suggest in chapter 5 that the practice of bloodletting may have played a part. We can be sure only of this: the consequences of this new belief were absolutely decisive. The theory of the *mo* not only justified, and in turn found justification in, therapies like moxibustion and needling, but it also illuminated, suddenly, connections between afflictions as seemingly disparate as shooting pains in the back and ringing in the ears. It provided, that is, a fresh framework for interpreting sickness. Henceforth the problem of understanding an illness became intimately linked to the task of determining the *mo* that governed it.

We return to the problem of diagnosis. English affords us little choice but to translate *mo* in two distinct ways. When referring to the objects of needling and moxibustion, we render *mo* as blood vessel, conduit, or the like; when the issue is diagnosis, we speak of the pulse. This is one legacy of Greek sphygmology — the bifurcation of the artery and the pulse, the structure and the motion. Lu Gwei-djen and Joseph Needham state flatly that the word *mo* had two meanings, and they even represent them with two separate Chinese characters.[82] But this obscures the guiding logic of Chinese palpation.

Qiemo began as and essentially remained exactly what its name

44

indicated: palpation of the various *mo*, that is, a procedure for tracking changes in the conduits that so powerfully affected the body's pains and powers. The *mo* grasped in diagnosis was the same *mo* burned and needled in therapy. *Qiemo* inquired not into the single voice that Greek doctors called *sphygmos*, but into a multiplicity of vital streams.

This is why doctors had to inspect twelve different sites — because there were, from the *Neijing* onward, twelve different *mo*. The *Lingshu*, the *Shanghanlun*, the *Jingui yaolue*, and the *Mojing* all preserve, in fact, vestiges of a diagnostic technique in which doctors examined twelve separate sites dispersed around the limbs, the trunk, the neck, and the head.[83] A floating quality at the ridge of the foot suggested an overactive stomach, while the same quality felt at the outer edge of the wrist bespoke intrusive wind. The meaning of the qualities discerned by the fingers changed with the place, because in the beginning distinct places belonged to and expressed distinct *mo*.

By the latter Han dynasty, admittedly, the *mo* were no longer independent tracts. The *Nanjing* links them together into one great circulation, and details how the *mo* moves three *cun* with each exhaling of breath, and three *cun* with each intake — six *cun* total with each respiratory cycle. A person takes 13,500 breaths in a day, and this translates into the *mo* making fifty circuits of the body. The *cunkou* inch-opening at the wrist represents the great confluence (*dahui*) of the *mo*, the site where circulation starts and ends — which is the reason, *Nanjing* 1 concludes, that doctors must inspect the *cunkou*.

The *Nanjing* was perhaps the first work to concentrate palpation exclusively on the wrist, and at the time of its composition this approach still needed justifying. As the very opening lines of the treatise explicitly acknowledge, "All the twelve conduits have *mo* which move (*dongmo*). Why, then, do you examine the *mo* at the *cunkou* alone to judge the five *zang* and six *fu*, life and death, prognoses auspicious and inauspicious?"

Conventional wisdom, the query implies, recognized twelve moving *mo*. At the end of the Han dynasty, people still knew the older, more laborious method of checking the various *mo* by palpating each one directly, at twelve widely separate sites in the body.

Nanjing 2 and 3 subdivide the *cunkou* into *cun*, *chi*, and *guan*, identifying the three as the realms, respectively, of the yang and the yin, and the divide between them. Interpretation here turned on relative position. Toward the head was yang, toward the feet was yin; toward the fingertips was yang, toward the trunk was yin; the surface was yang, the inner depths were yin. The *Suwen* method of interpreting the wrist, remember, linked the *cun* with the upper, or yang part of the body, the *chi* with the lower, or yin part of the body, and the *guan* with the viscera in between. *Nanjing* 18 would go further and associate the *cun*, *guan*, and *chi* with the heavenly, human, and earthly realms. Just as the microcosmic body reproduced the yin and yang dynamics of the macrocosm, so the yin and yang dynamics of the microcosmic body could in turn be shrunk to the inch-opening at the wrist. Topological analogy thus made it unnecessary to check from head to foot, and feeling the *mo* came to look like taking the pulse.

Appearances are deceptive, though. Unlike pulse taking, *qiemo* never aimed to judge the movements of arteries rooted in the heart. Although Han-dynasty doctors posited a continuous circulation and explored how they might alter one *mo* by treating another, this circulation had neither center nor starting point. There was a *mo* for the heart, but it claimed no special priority.[84] Glance at figure 4 and you see that the site for inspecting the heart was just one among twelve.

Each *mo* retained its own distinct dynamic. Early intuitions of a body organized into separate domains and ruled by separate *mo* were by no means obliterated by the rise of circulation theory. It was precisely because the *mo* didn't change uniformly and in unison that *qiemo* could tell the doctor which one to burn or needle.

To be sure, noting disparities among the various sites mattered more for acupuncture and moxibustion than for prescribing drugs. Case histories mostly just record the qualities discerned — "floating and slippery," say, or "sunken and weak" — without distinguishing between specific sites. Topological comparison wasn't always a priority.

Even so, belief in the profound meaningfulness of local difference never wavered. For the influential Li Gao (1180–1255), the *mo* at the left wrist thus revealed afflictions due to wind and cold and other noxious breaths invading from without, whereas inner deficiencies caused by faulty regimen appeared at the right wrist.[85] In the Ming dynasty, when Li Zhongzi (1588–1655) taught that the kidneys and stomach govern, respectively, prenatal and postnatal vitality, he also promoted diagnostic attention to the two sites on the foot which, in the ancient method of separately palpating each of the twelve *mo*, corresponded to the "moving *mo*" of these two viscera.[86] Whereas the pulse told a single story rooted in the heart, the revelations narrated by the *mo* were always subject, at least latently, to multiple local retellings.

But it wasn't just in their multiplicity that the *mo* differed from the pulse. Absent, too, from the conception of the *mo* was the Greek dichotomy of structure and function — the split between artery and pulse. The *Lingshu* declares: "That which dams up the nourishing *qi* and doesn't allow it to escape is called *mo*."[87] Says the *Suwen*: "*Mo* is the abode (*fu*) of the blood." Read by themselves, such passages invite us to imagine tubular conduits walling in vital fluids. We picture arteries and veins.

47

But the *Suwen* passage doesn't stop there:

> *Mo* is the abode of the blood. When it is long, then the *qi* is settled. When it is short, then the *qi* is ailing. When it is rapid, the heart is troubled. When it is large, then the ailment is progressing. When its upper part predominates, then the *qi* has risen. When its lower part predominates, then the *qi* is swollen. When it is intermittent, then the *qi* is debilitated. When it is thin, then *qi* is deficient. When it is rough, the heart aches.[88]

No sooner does "the abode of the blood" call blood vessels to mind, than adjectives like "settled," "rapid," and "intermittent" protest that no, what is really being discussed is the pulse. So it is misleading to assert, flatly, that the term *mo* had two meanings: the duality in English renderings is an artifact of translation. *Mo* were neither blood vessels nor the pulse, at least not as we conceive them, anatomically.

Just look at how they were grasped. Early on, in the treatise on the *mo* unearthed from the Zhangjiashan tombs, we find doctors focusing on six changes: whether the *mo* were full (*ying*) or empty (*xu*), quiet (*jing*) or moving (*dong*), slippery (*hua*), or rough (*se*).[89] How should *mo* be translated here? "Full" and "empty" could well characterize the contents of the artery, but "quiet" and "moving" appear to describe, contrarily, the activity of the pulse. And we simply wouldn't say, normally, of either the artery or the pulse, "It is slippery," or "It is rough." Yet in the art of *qiemo*, slipperiness and roughness ranked among the most privileged signs.

"In palpating the *chi* and the *cun*," observes *Suwen* treatise 5, "one checks whether the *mo* is floating (*fu*) or sunken (*chen*), slippery and rough, and knows the origin of the disease."[90] *Suwen* treatise 10 remarks similarly that if the five colors are what the eyes must diagnose, what the fingers must distinguish in the *mo* are the small and the large, the slippery and the rough, the floating and the sunken. The *Nanjing* replaces "small and large" with "long and short," but the other two contrasts remain: the floating versus the sunken, the slippery versus the rough.[91]

What made these distinctions so critical? They were by no means the only qualities sought out in *qiemo*; complete lists counted twenty-four or twenty-eight basic distinctions, or even more. Yet for some reason the medical classics singled out these four especially as signs framing the most vital confidences. To judge the bloom or withering of a person's life one had to inspect the *mo* and ask: Is it floating or sunken, slippery and rough? Why?

We must defer discussion of the first pair until chapter 4. The logic of the floating and the sunken takes us far beyond the imagination of the *mo* and engages the problem of the overall organization of life in the Chinese body. The interest in slipperiness and roughness, on the other hand, directly illuminates how feeling the *mo* differed, both in conception and in technique, from palpating the pulse.

If a slippery *mo* signaled wind (*feng*) afflictions, a rough *mo* bespoke paralysis (*bi*);[92] a slippery *mo* indicated slight fever, a rough *mo* slight cold;[93] a floating, slippery *mo* was typical of new diseases, a small, rough *mo* of chronic ailments;[94] a slippery *mo* meant superabundant yang breath, a rough *mo* excess yin blood.[95] These were some of the ways in which the slippery and the rough implied contrasting diagnoses. But for us the most interesting revelations reside rather in the contrast of their defining perceptions.

How did they differ, the slippery and the rough? The slippery *mo* "comes and goes in slippery flow, rolling rapidly, continuously forward" (*liuli zhanzhuan titiran*), says Wang Shuhe.[96] The rough *mo* is the opposite: it is "thin and slow, its movement is difficult

49

and dispersed, and sometimes it pauses, momentarily, before arriving";[97] one has the impression of flow made rough by resistance, struggling forward laboriously, instead of in a smooth, easy glide. "Like sawing bamboo," says the *Mojue*.[98]

Such descriptions speak to the central intuitions guiding Chinese palpation. The character *mo* (脈) combines the flesh radical (刖), marking a part of the body, with a pictograph (厎) for branching streams.[99] An early variant was composed with the sign for blood in place of the flesh radical — a variant which the *Shuowen jiezi* (ca. 100 C.E.), the first etymological dictionary in China, analyzes as the "branching flow of blood." We picture vital fluids streaming through the body.[100] Slipperiness and roughness mirrored the excessive fluency or faltering hesitations of its coursing.

Analogies between the earth's rivers and the currents of blood and breath in the body recur worldwide in the poetics of microcosm and macrocosm, and we encounter them more than once in writings of pre-Qin- and Han-dynasty China. The *Guanzi* thus calls water "the blood and breath of the earth,"[101] and the *Lingshu* more specifically pairs each of China's six major rivers with the six principal *mo* of the body.[102] Wang Chong (27–100?) explains: "The hundred rivers of the earth are like the streams of blood (*xuemo*) in man. Just as the streams of blood flow along, penetrating and spreading, and move and rest all according to their natural order, so it is with the hundred rivers. Their ebb and flow from dawn to dusk is like the expiration and inspiration of breath (*qi*)."[103]

Because of the familiarity of the trope, however, we may miss its special significance for palpation. And that is this: *mo* were more like rivers than conduits.[104] Their defining feature was flow. When Alfred Forke translated this paragraph, he succumbed to the spell of anatomy, and rendered *xuemo* as "blood vessels." But we are speaking of something that ebbs, spreads, and penetrates.

"Streams of blood" is surely the more natural, more exact translation here. *Xuemo* were the body's vital currents.

In medical texts the *mo* sometimes "moves" (*dong*) and only rarely "beats" (*bo*). Most often, it arrives (*lai*), departs (*qu*), travels (*xing*), and flows (*liu*).[105] Three *cun* with each inhaling of breath; three *cun* with every exhaling. The grammar of the term thus resists any facile identification of *mo* with blood vessels. But rendering *mo* as "pulse" is also awkward.

"The pulse," Charles Ozanam explained in his treatise on pulse physiology (1884), "is the movement of successive dilation and contraction that the wave of blood propelled by the systole of the heart imprints on the arterial tree."

> The essence of the pulse is thus not entirely the same as that of circulation. Circulation refers to the progress of the blood, the *materia progrediens*. The pulse is the form that this progression imprints on the walls of the blood vessels, the *forma materiae progredientis*.[106]

In its arrivals, departures, and travels, *mo* resembled circulation more than the pulse.

Instead of the vertical rise and fall of the arteries toward and away from the body surface, Chinese doctors sought to feel the horizontal streaming of the blood and breath parallel to the skin. The *Suwen* thus glosses slippery and rough in terms of the opposition of "following" (*cong*) and "resisting" (*ni*), and the *Lingshu* relates both pairs — slipperiness and roughness, and *cong* and *ni* — to the lessons of hydraulic engineering.[107] To *cong* was to be in the flow, or to go with the flow; to *ni* was to go against it. The eagerness to ascertain slipperiness or roughness mirrored the belief that life flowed.

Yet what does grasping flow really entail? How does the touch that tests the streaming of vitality differ from that which interrogates the pulsing artery? It is particularly with regard to this question of haptic style that the interest in slipperiness and roughness proves revealing. For doctors didn't seek these qualities in the *mo* alone. Early in the history of Chinese diagnostics they also found them in the *chi* — that is to say, in the skin of the inner forearm, near the elbow.

> The Yellow Emperor said to Qi Bo: "I wish to be able to name the sickness, to know what is happening inside by studying the outside; and I wish to do this without looking at facial color or feeling the *mo*, but through an examination of the *chi* alone. How do I do it?"
>
> Qi Bo replied: "You can determine the form of the illness by examining the *chi* to see if it is relaxed or tense, small or large, slippery or rough, and by feeling whether the flesh is firm or flabby.... If the skin of the *chi* is slippery, lustrous, oily, you are dealing with wind. If the skin of the *chi* is rough, you are dealing with wind-induced paralysis.[108]

Palpation of the forearm was once thought invaluable to understanding sickness. References to the technique appear throughout the *Neijing*, and we even find one treatise (*Lingshu*, treatise 74) devoted entirely to this form of diagnosis. Those who had mastered it could, just on the basis of that mastery alone, know "what was happening inside." So there were really *two* major forms of diagnostic touching in antiquity: besides the palpation of the *mo*, there was the palpation of the *chi*.

The two shared much in common. "I beg to ask," inquires the Yellow Emperor, "how the forms of sickness are related to whether the *mo* is relaxed or tense, small or large, slippery or rough" — thus naming exactly the same six qualities cited in the passage above as essential for diagnosing the forearm. Nor was this coincidence. Qualities in the *mo* and in the *chi* were comparable because they were regularly compared. Expounds Qi Bo:

> If the *mo* is tense, the skin of the *chi* is also tense. If the *mo* is relaxed, the skin of the *chi* is also relaxed. If the *mo* is small, the skin of the *chi* is also reduced and lacks *qi*. If the *mo* is large, the skin of the *chi* is also full, swelling. If the *mo* is slippery, the skin of the *chi* is also slippery. If the *mo* is rough, the skin of the *chi* is also rough.[109]

The two didn't, however, always change in unison. In fact, it was precisely because they often displayed completely disparate signs that comparing them was critical. If the conduits are full, for example, the *mo* is tense but the *chi* is relaxed.[110] The combination of a rough *chi* and a slippery *mo* announces much sweating. If the *chi* isn't hot, and the *mo* is slippery, the ailment is wind.[111] If the *chi* feels cold, and the *mo* is thin, this means diarrhea.[112]

The last two observations merit comment. Besides the six distinctions mentioned earlier, doctors also inspected whether the *chi* was hot or cold. *Lingshu* treatise 73 actually identifies these as two of the four elemental indications: by feeling whether the skin is cold or hot, slippery or rough, doctors can know where the disease lies.[113]

Now there is nothing unusual about noting the warmth or coolness of the skin. We can happen on these qualities even in the course of daily life — touching the arm of a lover, feeling the forehead of a child. The precepts of the *Suwen*, on the other hand, are rather more startling: it urges doctors to check for hot and cold at the *mokou* (= *cunkou*), the "mo-opening" at the wrist. Too little *qi* in the subsidiary channels and an excess of *qi* in the primary vessels manifests itself in a *mokou* that is hot, and a *chi* that is cold; if, contrarily, the main vessels fall depleted and the subsidiary

53

channels swell replete, the *chi* will be hot and full and the *mokou* cold and rough.[114] In short, doctors sought the same qualities in the wrist as in the forearm. The *mo* could be hot or cold, exactly like the skin of the inner arm.

In postclassical medicine, doctors seem to forget about diagnosing the *chi*. Not coincidentally, perhaps, they also cease to ask about hot and cold in the *mo*. (Of course, they continued routinely to infer chill and fever *in the body* from changes in the *mo*. But that is another matter: I speak here of feeling these qualities directly at the wrist itself.) Nonetheless, the fact that they once thought it meaningful and necessary to feel for the heat or coolness of the *mo* reminds us of the close kinship between Chinese "pulse taking" and palpation of the skin. *Qiemo* and the inspection of the *chi* were parallel forms of touching whose revelations were tightly entwined.

Judging slipperiness or roughness was basic to both. At times, one's fingers slide smoothly and effortlessly over the skin; at other times they catch and drag, and one has to pull them along, consciously. The similarities and linkage between the palpation of the *mo* and the diagnosis of the forearm intimates that the former may well have started as palpation *along* the *mo*, that in the beginning healers perhaps stroked the entire course of each *mo* to check, directly, the separate streams of a person's life.

People may lie, but the *mo* does not. The Emperor He (89–105 C.E.), the *History of the Later Han* records, wanted to test Guo Yu's skills,

> So he selected a catamite with very delicate hands and wrists and placed him behind a curtain alongside a girl, so that each put out one arm. He then had Yu examine the *mo* of both arms and asked him to identify the ailment of the "patient." Yu said, "The left arm is

54

yang and the right arm is yin. A *mo* is distinctly male or female. But this case would seem to be something different and your servant is puzzled as to why." The emperor sighed in admiration and praised his skill.[115]

The discovery that one could espy vital secrets about people merely by touching their wrists must once have seemed a marvel. Even now, when long familiarity has blunted our sense of wonder, and advanced imaging technologies have, at least in Western medicine, dramatically diminished its use, even now, we have but to track the changes at our own wrists to recover a sense of mystery.

Pictures from the past testify eloquently to the impact of this discovery. They remind us of how the art of palpation came to command the most absorbed concentration, the keenest curiosity, and how the art of healing became unthinkable without it (figures 5–8). They tell us little, though, about the inner content of this gesture, about how and what the fingers really knew.

Ancient Greek and Chinese doctors both fastened eventually on the wrist, which itself is noteworthy. There is, we've learned, nothing instinctive or obvious about the gesture; the worlds of knowledge that it opened up were unknown even to Hippocrates. Its common emergence in Greek and Chinese medicine, therefore, hints at latent affinities in the way the two traditions evolved.

Our present concern is with difference, however, and with the complexity of the act of touching. Two people can place their fingers on the "same" place and yet feel entirely different things. Where Greek doctors latched onto the pulse, Chinese doctors interrogated the *mo*. The divergence was as much a matter of experience as it was of theory. Greek and Chinese doctors *knew* the body differently because they *felt* it differently.

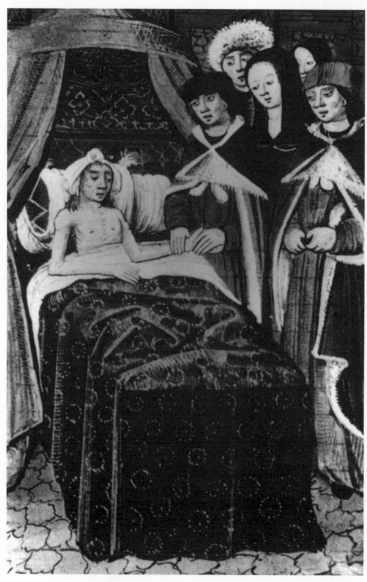

Figure 5. Medieval pulsetaking from Hunter MS.9, f.76, Wellcome Institute Library, London.

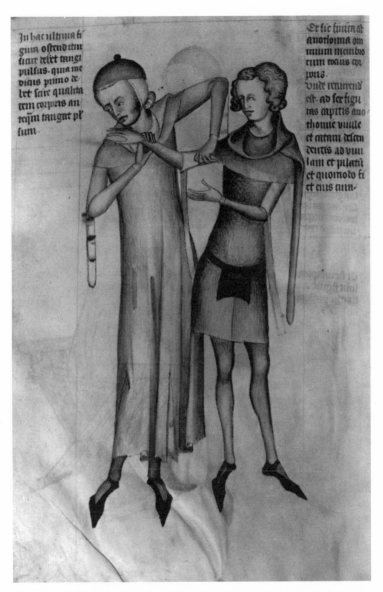

Figure 6. Medieval pulsetaking from Gui de Pavie, *Liber notabilium Philippi Septimi, francorum regis, a libris Galieni extractus* MS.334/569, fig. 18 (1345), Musée Condé, Chantilly (Lauros-Giraudon).

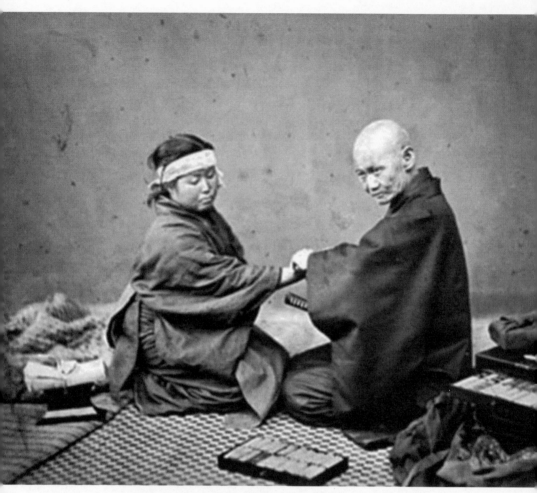
Figures 7 and 8. Pulsetaking in traditional Japan from the collection of the
International Research Center for Japanese Studies.

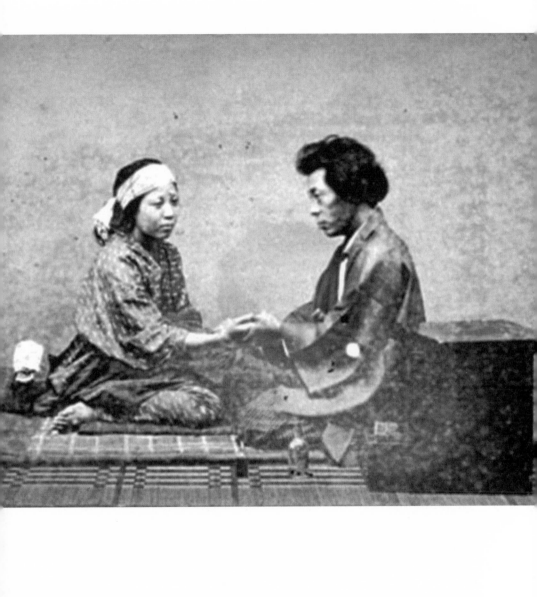

The converse also holds, of course. We could also say: they felt it differently because they knew it differently. My argument is not about precedence, but about interdependence. Theoretical preconceptions at once shaped and were shaped by the contours of haptic sensation. This is the primary lesson that I want to stress: when we study conceptions of the body, we are examining constructions not just in the mind, but also in the senses. Greek and Chinese doctors grasped the body differently — literally as well as figuratively. The puzzling otherness of medical traditions involves not least alternative styles of perceiving.

What goes into a perceptual style? This chapter has highlighted the influence of the presumed object of perception. We've learned that interpretations of the pulse and the *mo* entailed radically diverging expectations about what could and should be felt. But we have yet to consider another pivotal factor — an element absolutely fundamental to both thinking and feeling. I mean language. It is to the role and use of words that we now must turn.

CHAPTER TWO

The Expressiveness of Words

Chinese ideas about the pulse, opined J.J. Menuret de Chambaud (1733–1815), "are or appear to be very different from those of all other peoples."[1] While some Chinese pulses "quite conform with those that Galen established, and which all physicians recognize ... most are new to us, and appear very subtle and difficult to grasp."

> What relationship can there be, after all, between the beating of an artery and the movement of water sliding over a crack, a man undoing his belt, or someone wishing to wrap something up, but lacking the cloth to go all the way around?[2]

Chinese writings were rife with mystifying perceptions.

Yet in composing his article on pulse ("Pouls") for Diderot's *Encyclopédie*, Menuret de Chambaud felt unsure about how alien these perceptions really were. He knew that translations often blur, even distort, the outlines of feelings. So he wavered. After venturing initially that Chinese doctrines "are or *appear to be* very different," later in the article he ostensibly changed his mind. "The Chinese theory of the pulse," he concluded, "doesn't appear to diverge much from our ideas.... If some places jar our way of thinking, perhaps the failing is only in the terminology, and turn of expression, and should be attributed even more probably to the clumsiness of those who transmitted the feelings of the Chinese to us."[3]

This was likeliest — that the obscurity of what Chinese doctors wrote owed "chiefly to the way in which they express[ed] themselves, their little-understood allegorical style."[4] Chances were that Chinese texts echoed familiar truths, but in an unfamiliar voice.

Earlier in the century, John Floyer proffered a crisper view. He discerned in Chinese pulse writings the voice of an alternative mindset. "Europeans excel in reasoning and judgment, and clearness of expression," he suggested, whereas "Asiatics have a gay luxurious imagination."[5] Styles of writing mirrored styles of thinking. Europeans prized sober rational precision; the Chinese were fanciful and poetic.

Floyer took for granted that sober reason was to be preferred, but he didn't for all that dismiss Chinese teachings as delusions. No, witnesses in China had convinced him of the wonderful local "skill in pulses." Reading about Chinese doctrines, Floyer thus found "good sense, tho' express'd in the Asiatic way, whose words are sorts of hieroglyphicks, as well as their characters; and their expressions are fitter for poetry and oratory, than philosophy."[6] In accusing the imagination, he wasn't so much scoffing superciliously as struggling to figure, like Menuret de Chambaud, why writings that should have illumined secrets instead posed puzzles.

Floyer reasoned: Chinese doctors enjoyed the wisdom of "curious experience, examined and approved for four thousand years."[7] Through millennia of careful observation they had accumulated real knowledge about the body; their practical success in diagnosing and curing was proof. If, therefore, their texts appeared inscrutable and bizarre, the problem had to lie not in the knowledge itself, but in its formulation, its refraction through "luxurious imagination." Chinese doctors knew authentic truths, but in some unknown, exotic way.

Was his analysis right? What does style signify in the end? What does the manner in which people speak tell us about how and what they know? The oddity of Chinese descriptions *seemed* to reveal the oddity of Chinese perceptions, but it was possibly just the words that threw one off. For Menuret de Chambaud, for John Floyer, the sole certainty was the queer, perplexing otherness of Chinese "allegorical" discourse. The strange voice.

There is a gap between touching and feeling. Perceptions aren't raw experiences. What we perceive, when we touch something, depends largely on *how* we touch it — whether we place our hands gingerly, or grip hard, whether our fingers explore with care, or merely tap impatiently. But how we handle an object depends, in turn, on how we conceive it. The delicacy with which we hold antique china disappears when we pick up modern plastic imitations. The manner in which we cradle the face of a loved one is worlds apart from our touch when we brush, involuntarily, against someone we despise or fear.

Part of the foreignness of Chinese writings can be explained thus. The *mo* and the pulse, chapter 1 revealed, were grasped differently — under the fingers, and in the mind. Menuret de Chambaud's first impression was right: many Chinese distinctions *were* new. Doctors in China detected slipperiness and roughness where Greek pulse takers did not, because feeling the *mo* meant feeling something that flowed. Conversely, traits that Herophilus and Galen found so revealing in the pulse's message — rhythm, for instance — regularly went unnamed and unrecognized (and would have scarcely made sense) in *qiemo*, for they presupposed a picture of the pulsating artery. Mutually unfamiliar words named mutually unfamiliar perceptions.

But by itself this explanation is too simple. It ignores, to begin, how language itself sculpts perceptions, how words shape, at the same time as they label, what the fingers feel. A diagnostic system that speaks only of "hard" and "soft" trains the hand only to separate the hard from the soft. A discourse that further splices "tense" from "hard," "slack" from "weak," fosters a finer tact.

And in any case, the problem of language and perception goes deeper than local idiosyncrasies of vocabulary, than Chinese or European sensitivity or insensitivity to particular qualities. Besides using different words, diagnosticians in China and Europe also and more fundamentally *used words differently*. It is especially this contrast in usage that I wish to explore — how styles of speaking relate to styles of knowing.

John Floyer saw reason and judgment mirrored in European clearness, and he contrasted these to the play, in China, of gay, luxurious imagination. But clearness, in Europe, was less a characteristic trait than a characteristic ideal, less a fact than a desire. Historically, what marked Western discourse on the pulse was above all the fierce *yearning* for clarity. When Floyer and Menuret de Chambaud called the Chinese style imaginative and allegorical, they betrayed in part their wonder at a people apparently free of this longing — a culture curiously indifferent to, perhaps even ignorant of, the hunger for transparency.

Nothing forces us now, however, to treat this hunger as any less strange than its lack. The question of diverging styles isn't a problem of one-sided (i.e., Chinese) peculiarity; the compulsion to clarify is itself an enigma. What's more, this enigma lies at the core of one of the most remarkable features of pulse knowledge. I mean its slender fragility.

The Fragility of Haptic Knowledge

Consider how knowing the *mo* remains crucial, even today, to knowing the body. Consider how practitioners of traditional Chinese medicine still consult classics like the *Mojing*, in the original and in modern synopses, for clinical guidance. Consider that *qiemo* is still very much alive.

And then consider how pulse taking in Western medicine barely survives, how it has become a shriveled, meager science — mostly the bare counting of beats. Doctors now seek the essence of the heart's speech in machines, which translate it into graphs and numbers, rather than under the fingers, in haptic knowledge. Classical tomes on the training of the touch gather dust, as antiquated lore.

What should we make of this contrast? Superficially, the question may appear trivial. Traditional Chinese medicine is traditional, after all — that is, pretechnological — whereas contemporary Western medicine decidedly is not. The decline of diagnostic touching in the West seems almost an inevitable, natural consequence of the rise of modern technology. We readily suppose the precision and objectivity of machines making human touch look hopelessly obtuse and unreliable.[8]

But this interpretation reverses the historical order of things. Doubts about pulse diagnosis in fact predated — and indeed helped spur the invention of — machines like the sphygmograph and the EKG. The separate fates of *qiemo* and pulse taking have deeper roots than the divide between traditional and technological approaches to medicine.

Chapter 1 cited European and American doctors proclaiming the indispensability of pulse study; it would be easy to quote others. Read in context, however, such pronouncements often seem more defensive than celebratory, prefacing attempts to revive an art in decline, reclaim lost wisdom. Henri Fouquet's pulse treatise

65

of 1767 thus opens by confidently declaring, "Doctors agree that the most useful of all the forms of knowledge governing medicine is knowledge of the pulse." But Fouquet then immediately adds, "Nevertheless, it appears — and one cannot but note this with surprise — that this branch of the art has advanced very little for several centuries. Indeed, the study of the pulse has been long neglected...."[9]

Fouquet's contemporary Théophile de Bordeu even speaks of classical pulse doctrines as having "slipped into oblivion";[10] and James Nihell begins his study of the pulse by conceding that the art about which he proposed to write was "so little thought of" that it had "long fallen into discredit."[11] Centuries before their time, faith in the pulse had already faltered.

Why? A chronic concern was the idiosyncrasy of perceptions: people don't all feel things in the same way. An expert detects an "antcrawling" pulse where a beginner finds nothing unusual. Who is right? The discrepancy may well lie in the beginner's blunt tact. Then again, the alleged expert may be lying.

Or hallucinating. Despite trying for months, the eighteenth-century physician Duchemin de l'Etang still couldn't distinguish the pulses named by the self-proclaimed experts of his day. "It was from that moment," he recounts, "that I began to suspect that there might be a bit of enthusiasm and imagination behind the whole matter."[12] When others claimed to perceive what he couldn't, perhaps they were really fooling themselves. Perhaps the dazzling fabric of sphygmological revelation was spun from threads of self-deception, like the emperor's new clothes.

Specific ideas, like the image of the pulsing artery, can shape what the fingers feel. But no less influential are broad attitudes, such as trust and suspicion. "The more information a physician expects to obtain from the pulse," remarked Milo North in 1826, "the more light he will receive."

66

And it appears to me equally plain that when a man feels uncertainty whether much dependence can be placed upon it, he must remain totally unacquainted with the nature of its communications. I cannot but think that it is this scepticism, more than any organic defect of touch or want of definite terms, which has rendered it fashionable to speak lightly of the indications of the pulse.[13]

Most pulses aren't plain and unmistakable, and one must learn to feel them. Yet if one suspects from the start that there is nothing to be learned, then indeed one may learn nothing. When the English doctor Richard Burke couldn't discern what others described, he soon gave up trying, persuading himself "that writers [on the pulse]...have refined too much, and that after all the pulse is not so very important as some would have us believe."[14] Pulse knowledge was exquisitely vulnerable to doubt.

Can such doubt be resolved? Sphygmologists all allowed that some people may be more sensitive than others, and that training is essential. But for such training even to become possible, one must be able to say, precisely and unambiguously, what the fingers should feel. Time and again, critics and defenders of pulse diagnosis alike returned to this as the real crux: to teach or learn the varieties of pulses one needs clear words. Yet clarity proved ever elusive.

You open Galen's treatises on the pulse expecting to learn how Greek doctors interpreted the pulse, and you are soon at sea. For you find yourself reading more about semantics than about semiology, more about the definition of words, than about the recognition of diseases. Hundreds upon hundreds of pages devoted to fixing, refining, explicating the sense of terms. What is really meant, Galen asks, by a "strong pulse" or a "large pulse"? How does one separate "fast" from "frequent"?

Modern scholars have judged these pages almost unbearably tedious. "The most uncongenial of all to read," sighs Vivian Nutton; "Galen at his pettifogging worst," C.R.S. Harris complains.[15] Still, there is no mistaking Galen's earnestness; for him, a true science of the pulse stood or fell with the exact use of exact words. The hunger for lucidity was ancient.

We can imagine numerous factors contributing to this hunger. The multiplicity of Mediterranean tongues, for instance. Galen laments: doctors living in disparate places and speaking different dialects not only name pulses differently, but compound the confusion by their parochial pride — their insistence on local usage, and their derision of foreign terms.[16] Another, still more powerful influence was the philosophical tradition descending from Socrates through Plato, which placed such ardent emphasis on definition; a tradition itself associated with the popularity, in Greek society more generally, of public debate and disputation. Galen's own time saw a renewed vogue of sophists and rhetoricians, the flourishing of the Second Sophistic, when ties between medicine, philosophy, and rhetoric became tighter than ever. Aelius Aristides thus characterizes Galen's teacher Satyrus as both doctor and sophist. "Doctor-sophist" (*iatrosophistos*) and "doctor-philosopher" (*iatrophilosophos*) were common professional titles.[17]

Yet by themselves, explanations of Galen's context can't suffice. The yearning for clearness possessed Western pulse takers far beyond the polyglot Mediterranean and long after the Second Sophistic. If Galen attacked the sloppy language of his predecessors, Josephus Struthius in the sixteenth century denounced Galen's own treatises for being so convoluted that "hardly one in a thousand might understand them."[18] Eighteenth-century physicians, too, condemned Galen's language. It was chiefly against his vocabulary, Théophile de Bordeu (1722–76) relates, and especially his use of fanciful metaphors — labeling pulses with such names as the "antcrawling," the "mouselike," and the "gazelling" — that modern students of the pulse had rebelled.[19]

The eventual push to distill pulse taking to beat counting represented the culmination of this ancient quest for transparency. The obstacles blocking a reliable science of the pulse, urged William Heberden, went beyond fanciful metaphors. Addressing the Royal College of Physicians in 1772, Heberden declared it "highly unlikely" that *any* of the terms used to qualify the pulse "are perfectly understood or applied by all to the same sensations and have in everyone's mind the same meaning." He advised doctors, therefore, to attend

> more to such circumstances of the pulse in which they could neither mistake nor be misunderstood. Fortunately, there is one of this sort, which not only on this account, but likewise for its importance deserves all our attention. What I mean is, the frequency or quickness of the pulse.... This is the same in all parts of the body, and cannot be affected by the constitutional firmness or flaccidity, or smallness or largeness of the artery, or by its lying deeper or more superficially; and is capable of being numbered, and consequently of being most perfectly described and communicated to others.[20]

Should doctors be swayed in what they diagnose by what they can, or can't, communicate? Heberden's reasoning calls to mind the story of the man who, having lost his wallet in a dark lane, searches for it in the adjacent avenue because of the better lighting. Still, his approach was seductive. Pulse rates remain identical no matter who checks, which artery one presses, how one grasps it. Just as importantly, misunderstandings can't arise. Eighty-two. Ninety-five. One hundred and seven. Unlike metaphors such as the "anting" or "worming," unlike even plain adjectives like "hard" and "soft," numbers suffer no semantic slack.

The proposal was radical only in its solution, in the way it suddenly stripped the pulse's message to bare numerals alone; it was eminently traditional in its conception of the problem, its motivating intuitions. Indeed, it represented a logical conclusion — the mechanical sphygmograph would later be another — to a tradition that had long identified the quest for a secure science of the pulse with the challenge of eradicating the betrayals of language. Like many before him, Heberden was convinced that "the chief source of confusion is the employment of terms which are susceptible to more than one interpretation."[21] Numbers promised absolute clarity.

Why did pulse takers keep blaming language for the uncertainties of the fingers and the mind? The question is critical to looking afresh and comparatively at the enterprise of pulse diagnosis. For nothing more distinctly characterized the history of discourse on the pulse than this nervousness about words. We encounter it time and again — the haunting sense that vague terms are blunting, distorting, and misrepresenting what the fingers feel, the restless urge to rename and redefine, the ever-renewed hope that this time one might get it right. As if the failures securely to grasp the pulse were really just failures properly to name and describe it. As if the problem of knowledge was, at its heart, a problem of words.

The vocabulary of *qiemo* inspired no such anxieties, and its terminology remained more stable. Of the twenty-four *mo* identified by the *Mojing* — the basic vocabulary of the language of life — at least fourteen were already known to Chunyu Yi in the early second century B.C.E., and all were current by the time of the *Neijing*. Over the course of two millennia, physicians ventured a few additions, expanding the lexicon to twenty-eight, even thirty-two terms;[22] but these were accretions on a canonical core. Unlike in Europe, the history of palpation in China witnessed no calls for clearer language, no disputes over definitions, no gnawing doubts about whether people all named the same perceptions when they uttered the same words.

Doctors clasped the *mo* with startling confidence. Overconfidence, even. If pulse takers in Europe lamented periodically that palpation wasn't heeded enough, their Chinese counterparts decried rather the habit of relying too much on the touch and neglecting the other senses. Shi Fa's *Chabing zhinan* (1241) echoed a common charge: "The study of medicine is all contained in the divine, the sagely, the crafty, and the skillful. But doctors today commonly leave out three of these and focus on one. Which one? 'To touch and know is called skillful.' Rather than deploy this expression in its true sense, however, they use it by itself, out of context, and thus deceive the world."[23]

Palpation was just one, and the lowliest, of four ways to know the body — theoretically. Diagnosis encompassed the "divine" art of gazing, the "sagely" art of listening and smelling, the "crafty" art of questioning, and the "skillful" art of touching. Someone who learned the last thus qualified only as skillful, while those who mastered hearing and seeing achieved sageliness and divinity. In practice, however, doctors made a regular fetish of palpation and, worse, brazenly paraded their bias as a special virtue.

Here is the paradox of *qiemo*. Unlike pulse taking in the West, palpation in China was practiced confidently and flourished stably for over two thousand years, and still flourishes today. Yet its language was precisely of the sort that Western pulse takers strove so strenuously to expunge, abounding in the poetic, "imaginative" speech that they believed fatal to a secure science. Stranger still, Chinese doctors themselves freely acknowledged the fluid subtlety of the *mo*, the bluntness of the touch, and the inadequacy of words. Qualities like "the chordlike and the tense, the floating and the hollow," declared the preface of the *Mojing*, "all blend into one another and are closely related."[24] Differing merely by slight shades of feeling, the various *mo* are hard to separate, readily muddled. For diagnosticians of later ages this would be a commonplace. Summarizing accepted wisdom, Li Zhongzi mused in the seventeenth-century:

> The subtlety of the principles of the *mo* has been noted since antiquity. In the past there was the Yellow Emperor, who displayed divine intelligence from the moment he was born. Yet even he likened [grasping these principles] to peering into a profound abyss and coming up against floating clouds. Xu Shuwei said, "The principles of the *mo* are mysterious and hard to clarify. What my mind can comprehend my mouth cannot transmit." All that can be noted with brush and ink and all that be expressed with the mouth and tongue are but traces and likenesses (*jixiang*).[25]

Where European sphygmologists worried chiefly about misnomers and misconstruals — about misuses of language, which, as misuses, could theoretically be rectified — Li Zhongzi here affirmed more unbudging limits. It was in the very nature of language and the *mo* that words should fall short. The *mo* was inevitably mysterious, ineffable.

Li believed that this was why classical descriptions of the *mo* were typically so roundabout and allusive — why the slippery *mo* had to be likened to a "smooth succession of rolling pearls" and the rough *mo* to "rain-soaked sand." Reality always lay beyond the "traces and likenesses." Ancient authors didn't seek deliberately to be cryptic, they tried to communicate their insights. The words just never sufficed.[26]

How can we reconcile this view of words as mere "traces and likenesses" with their stable and confident use over millennia? Why wasn't the language of *qiemo* subject, like that of pulse diagnosis, to constant criticism and revision?

The Daoist overtones of Li Zhongzi's reference to floating clouds and dark ravines hint at the possibility that stability here reflected more resignation than trust: perhaps doctors in China didn't search for clearer terms because they believed that simulacra, vague likenesses, were all that could be hoped for. Perhaps they assumed from the start that complete clarity lay beyond reach. The opening rhapsody of Laozi's *Daodejing* — "The Way that can be named is not the eternal Way; the Name that can be named is not the eternal Name" — was but the most celebrated utterance of the belief, often echoed in later writings, that sublime truths defied articulation. To name, Zhuangzi likewise taught, is to impose distinctions on what naturally has no seams, to carve up and ruin the unspeakable integrity of the world.[27]

Yet this was by no means the sole, or even dominant view of language. Official state orthodoxy, for its part, vigorously championed linguistic precision as a cornerstone of social order. When words lose their customary meanings, Confucian thinkers urged, when they are applied recklessly to realities to which they weren't intended to apply, moral judgment melts away. Opportunists relabel bandits as kings and altruism as foolishness; sophists deviously twist meanings to make betrayal appear praiseworthy and recast righteousness as treachery. It is in this way that people lose their compass of superior and inferior, right and wrong, and chaos prevails.[28] Indiscriminate language spawns wanton indiscrimination. So the *Book of Rites* enjoined death for those who subverted the legal order by sophistical hairsplitting and changing the names of things.[29]

The attitudes of doctors were almost certainly closer to the

Confucian perspective than to the Daoist, and this not because the former exercised greater influence on medicine — overall, in my view, rather the reverse held true — but because of the exigencies of practical action. The management of the body, like the ordering of the state, required firm distinctions. Especially in *qiemo*. Semantically and perceptually, the chordlike *mo* and the tense *mo* might deviate merely by the finest shades, but the practical consequences of the two, the diagnoses and cures they implied, were totally distinct. Resignation to ambiguity was a luxury medicine couldn't afford. Whether a patient found relief and recovered, or suffered greater agonies, or died — all this depended on doctors making the right discriminations, seizing the exact nuance.

So in China, as in Europe, accurate names were indispensable to the art of healing. If the vocabulary of *qiemo* escaped the fitful doubting that proved so corrosive to pulse diagnosis, it wasn't because Chinese doctors felt no need for exactness, or were resigned to stunted communication. Their confidence in words requires other explanations.

Distinguished scholars have pointed out, of course, that Western intellectual life was marked by more vigorous and radical debate than can be found in China, whereas Chinese thinkers tended to place greater weight on canonical texts and authorities.[30] Viewed against this backdrop, the stable transmission of the classical language of palpation seems almost predictable — another instance of a familiar pattern, further proof of the irenic traditionalism running through all of Chinese medicine.

Yet in the end, such generalities teach us little about the problem at hand. A diagnostic vocabulary, after all, can't be sustained by faith alone, nor can its fate be settled by decree. Terms persist and prosper only as long as people can use them. Even if doctors a thousand years after the *Mojing* trusted the authority of canonical terms, they still had to make these terms work for them, practically, in the treatment of the sick; they had to feel that the terminology forged by others in remote antiquity effectively captured and communicated what they themselves experienced under their fingers, here and now. And somehow they did — appropriating ancient terms confidently and consistently for two millennia, untroubled by the demons that haunted the European pulse taker, innocent of suspicions about knowledge betrayed by words.

This is the puzzle. Writings on *qiemo* emphasized on the one hand that fine distinctions were indispensable to accurate diagnosis, and conceded on the other that language offers no more than vague "traces and likenesses." We would have expected this combination to condemn palpation to failure, or at least perpetual instability; but it didn't. Doctors carried on unfazed.

How did they do it? Why didn't the awareness of traces and similarities engender in *qiemo* an unquenchable thirst for clarity like that which so decisively shaped European pulse taking? To answer this question we need first to analyze more carefully the nature of this thirst in Europe. We must begin by pondering just how lucid description differs from the obscure.

The Quest for Clarity

What separates the language of exact judgment from that of extravagant imagination?

Eighteenth-century pulse takers explained: it is chiefly a matter of literal versus figurative speech. Only the former can insure limpid understanding; the latter is profoundly unreliable. Fanciful figures were the downfall of Galen's sphygmology, the principal reason why the moderns had abandoned it. Terms such as the "gazelling," the "anting," and the "worming," which likened pulse motions to the movements of animals, were simply too whimsical, too inexact. So they said.

75

Perhaps the criticism was unfair — such poetic nomenclature actually formed only a minor, exceptional part of Galenic pulse writings. Certainly it was ironic. Galen himself had already denounced figuralism, and just as vigorously as his later critics. He, too, sought clarity through literalness.

"If ever we have literal names," Galen urged (and, he says elsewhere, "in the case of touch, all [qualities] have been named"), "it is always fitting to use them."

> But if not, it is always more fitting to explain each [nameless] thing by means of a *logos* [a reasoned account], and not to name them on the basis of metaphor.... The initial instruction of all scientific matters, however, requires literal words, for the sake of it [scientific instruction] being both clear and distinctly articulated.[31]

Clarity and distinct articulation were the goals, and literalness the necessary means. Habitually, names were applied too loosely. Inexactness crept in through metaphor: words were displaced from their proper sense and transferred to remote matters. Yes, figurative speech had its uses. It could occasionally help, for instance, to evoke things that have no name, such as certain smells.[32] Still, for science, this rule was basic: literalness first and foremost.

How do we separate, though, the proper, literal deployment of a word from the figurative uses? Textbooks typically make the task sound easy. We point at an apple tree and say, "The apples aren't ripe yet"; this is the literal use of the word "apples." When we observe "That son is the apple of her eye," we speak metaphorically.

Suppose, though, that a doctor feels a patient's wrist and asserts, "This is a rough pulse." Is "rough" here literal or figurative?

Consider two other usages. You slide your fingertips over sandpaper and confirm, "Yes, this surface is rough." Another time, you trudge wearily home, toss down your briefcase, and sigh, "I've had a rough day!" Most of us would probably say: the first "rough" is literal, the second figurative — the difference presumably being that roughness is intrinsic to the sandpaper, whereas the roughness of a day resides in our perception of it. In the former, that is, roughness belongs to the object, whereas in the latter, it describes our subjective experience. The literal or figurative status of the "rough pulse" thus seems to turn on this: whether we believe that roughness can inhere in the pulse itself, or think that "rough" names only how the pulse *appears* to us.

The answer isn't obvious. Scrutinized philosophically, the line demarcating objective traits from subjective perceptions readily blurs, even fades. Not a few thinkers have argued that *all* qualities, including the roughness of sandpaper and the redness of cherries, hinge on human judgment. Nonetheless, the fact remains that, historically, pulse takers absolutely insisted on the demarcation. This is the lesson to remember.

For it explains why European readers of the *Mojue* felt so unsettled by, and dissatisfied with, the Chinese "allegorical style." What is a rough *mo*? Doctors in China seemed content to say, "It is like sawing bamboo," or "It is like rain-soaked sand." To Western pulse takers, these didn't count as answers. Their very form was wrong: they spoke only of how someone might imagine a rough *mo*, and said nothing about what a rough *mo* actually *is*.

Jumbling facts and perceptions, however, was a failing to which many were apparently prone. French and English theorists, complained a doctor in 1832, had spliced the pulse so finely, "and rendered its variations numerous and complicated, as almost to defy comprehension. Heberden remarks, 'such minute distinctions of the several pulses exist chiefly in the imagination of the makers, or at least have little place in the knowledge and cure of diseases.' Dr. Hunter could never feel the nice distinctions in the pulse that many others did, and ... [he] held that the nicer peculiarities in the pulse are only sensations in the mind."[33]

Distinctions existing "chiefly in the imagination," "only sensations in the mind." Such phrases tell of a belief in distinctions other than those forged in the imagination; they presume the existence of qualities in reality itself, out there, already given, waiting to be felt. Besides sensations in the mind, there had to be sensations under the fingers, qualities known directly and immediately, rather than inferred, projected, filtered through distorting subjectivity. These were the traits that words had to convey with unadorned literalness.

The crucial divide, then, lay between a world of perceptions and a world of facts. Concretely, for Galen the primary facts of the pulse were the generic categories of size, speed, frequency, and rhythm, and the modulations that articulated them, such as large and small, fast and slow, frequent and rare. Size spoke to the magnitude of the artery's dilation; speed named how quickly, or slowly, this expansion occurred; frequency measured the interval between successive dilations; rhythm compared the artery's dilation to its contraction. These facts all shared one feature: they were all realities subject to precise, geometrical analysis. Galen thus posited twenty-seven variations in size, visualizing an artery's length, breadth, and height, and reasoning that the pulsatile expansion along each of these three dimensions could be large, or small, or in-between, making for twenty-seven combinations. Here, in the image of the pulsing blood vessel beheld vividly in the mind's eye, was the pulse as pure fact — the proper object of clear, literal knowledge.

Undergirding the ideal of literal clarity about the pulse was thus a conception of objectivity defined importantly by habits of picturing. And therein lay its fragility. For some aspects of the pulse defied ready visualization. Qualities such as strong and weak, full and empty, hard and soft, for example. The fingers had some-how to grasp these directly.

Strength and fullness proved especially controversial. Magnus rejected strength as an elementary category, arguing that it was really a composite of size, speed, and fullness.[34] Archigenes countered that strength was an independent quality, corresponding to the degree of pneumatic tone (*tonos*). Galen, in turn, faulted Archigenes for confusing the cause of a strong pulse with its definition — explaining why a pulse feels strong, Galen insisted, isn't at all the same as defining what a strong pulse is.[35]

As for fullness, Herophilus apparently hadn't recognized it. By Galen's time, however, doctors were wrestling with the issue of whether "full" and "empty" referred to the body of the artery or to its contents, and if to its contents, whether to quantity or qual-ity — struggling to fix the objective fact beneath the perception.[36] Galen himself dropped the category, and spoke only of hardness and softness, the consistency of the arterial wall. In this way, aspects of touch irreducible to the image of the artery and its motions were perpetually unstable, subject to reinterpretation. Qualities such as strong, full, and tense were hard to picture, and hence, hard to define.

Discourse on the pulse, in short, bound the understanding of meanings inseparably to the picturing of images. Inveighing against the hairsplitting of sophists — who, he quips, can't even buy veg-etables without definitions — Galen repeats over and again that he cares not at all about the name (*onoma*), but only about the thing or fact (*pragma*) that it identifies.[37] In a sense, words don't mat-ter, they are just conventional labels.

At other times, however, Galen resorts to a slightly different formula. He has one concern alone, he stresses: "to know the idea underlying what is said" (*ton noun tou legomenou*). Haggling over words is pointless because a word merely stands in for a *nous* or an *ennoia* — a thought or an idea. It is the thought that counts.[38]

Logically, these aren't at all the same — a thing and the idea of the thing. Yet in sphygmology, the elision of *pragma* and *ennoia* easily passed unnoticed. On the one hand, the etymologies of the Greek terms *nous*, *ennoia*, and *idea* all associated thoughts with mental pictures. On the other hand, the clearest, most securely objective aspects of the pulse derived their clarity and objectivity from the possibility of picturing them. So in practice the line between the *ennoia* of a broad pulse, say, and the *pragma* of a broad pulse was negligibly thin. The thought and the reality alike were anchored in the imagining of the artery's lateral spread.

"The pulse can only be known by the touch," Théophile de Bordeu would later declare. One knows it by experience and not by reasoning, in much the same way that one comes to know colors, or movement, or sound, or heat. Nonetheless, even he couldn't deny the claims of visualization. "It is only by palpating that one can have an idea of it, and form an image of it." Knowing was a sort of inner seeing. Hence the importance of knowing "the anatomy of the parts whose oscillations constitute the pulse ... in order to have clear notions (*notions claires*) about the nature of the pulse."[39]

What underlay the restless push in Western sphygmology for ever more perspicuous words? Partly, I've suggested, it was fueled by qualities such as strong and tense, which, because they defied lucid picturing, eluded sharp and stable definition. But ultimately, the problem went deeper. Heberden, remember, eventually cast doubt on all words. The core problem lay in the human inability to see the imaginings of others.

Listening to a doctor who reports an undulating pulse, we may strain to visualize the fact conveyed by the word. We ask, "What exactly do you mean by that?" struggling to "make clear" in our minds the image motivating the speaker. Yet we can never be fully confident about our insights, never be sure of the coincidence of imaginings. Once speaking is conceived as the expression of ideas in the mind, then the hunger for transparency becomes irresistible — though it remains ever insatiable, though we cannot peer into other minds. Does your idea of "undulating" correspond to mine? We simply cannot know.

Rhythm

Exasperated at the obscurity of Galen's writings, "which no reader of the Latin text would understand even if he worked on them till he became crazy," the Polish doctor Josephus Struthius (1510–68) tried to represent the pulse without words, relying instead on limpid musical notes to communicate the varieties of its rhythms.[40] In the next century, Samuel Hafenreffer's *Monochordon symbolico-biomanticum* (1640) and Athanasius Kircher's *Musurgia universalis* (1650) carried this initiative further and translated all the major pulses into music; and in 1769, François Nicolas Marquet composed the most elaborate renditions of all, weaving for instance the beats of a healthy pulse into the measures of a minuet (figures 9–12).[41] Visual renderings of the pulse in early modern Europe thus assumed a form quite different from Shi Fa's pictures of the *mo* (figure 13). Prior to the invention of the sphygmograph in the mid-nineteenth century, the favored transcriptions were musical.

Struthius may have invented the method, but the intuitions underlying such transcriptions of the pulse had a long history. The great medieval authority Avicenna (Ibn Sīna, 980–1037), for instance, insisted already that only the musically trained could truly know the pulse — because "the pulse is of a musical nature":

> [T]hat is to say, it resembles aspects of which the science of music consists: pulse beats are comparable to rhythmic beats as regards

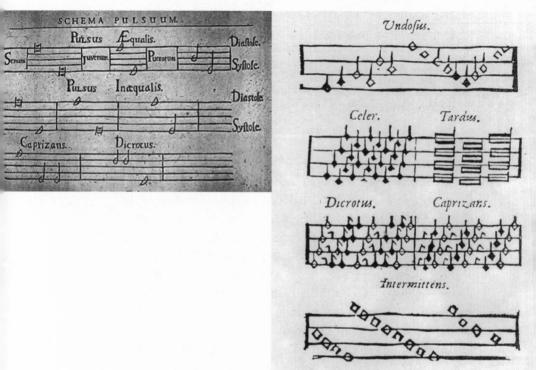

Figure 9. Josephus Struthius, *Ars sphygmica*, Noma Research Archives for Science and Medicine, Tokyo.

Figure 10. Samuel Hafenreffer, *Monochordon symbolico-biomanticum* (Ulm, 1640), National Library of Medicine.

Figure 11. Athanasius Kircher, *Musurgia universalis* (Rome, 1650), National Library of Medicine.

Figure 12. François Nicolas Marquet, *Nouvelle méthode facile et curieuse, pour connaître le pouls par les notes de la musique* (Amsterdam, 1769), National Library of Medicine.

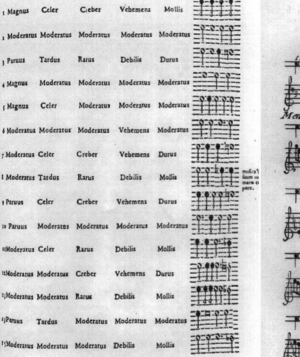

1 Magnus	Celer	Creber	Vehemens	Mollis
2 Moderatus	Moderatus	Moderatus	Moderatus	Moderatus
3 Paruus	Tardus	Rarus	Debilis	Durus
4 Magnus	Moderatus	Moderatus	Moderatus	Moderatus
5 Magnus	Celer	Moderatus	Moderatus	Moderatus
6 Moderatus	Moderatus	Moderatus	Vehemens	Moderatus
7 Moderatus	Celer	Creber	Vehemens	Durus
8 Moderatus	Tardus	Rarus	Debilis	Mollis
9 Paruus	Celer	Creber	Vehemens	Durus
10 Paruus	Moderatus	Moderatus	Moderatus	Moderatus
11 Moderatus	Celer	Rarus	Debilis	Mollis
12 Moderatus	Moderatus	Creber	Vehemens	Durus
13 Moderatus	Moderatus	Rarus	Debilis	Mollis
14 Paruus	Tardus	Moderatus	Moderatus	Moderatus
15 Moderatus	Moderatus	Moderatus	Debilis	Mollis

musica?
suum m
mare c
pore.

Atque

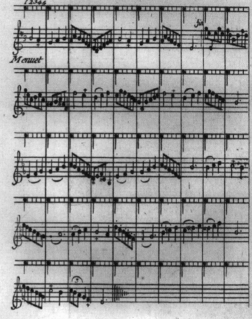

Exemple du Poulx naturel reglé

Menuet

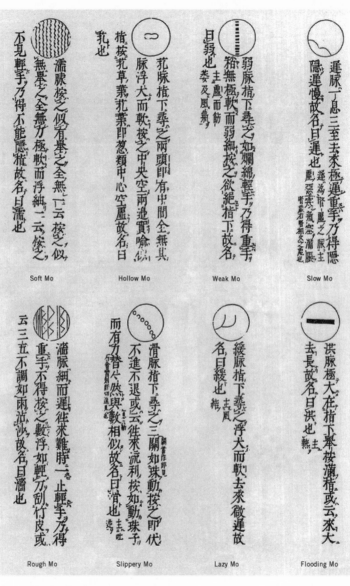

Figure 13. Shi Fa, *Chabing zhinan*, Fujikawa Collection, Kyoto University Library.

both speed and frequency; the qualities of pulse beats, namely, strength, weakness, and the extent of the artery's expansion, are comparable to the qualities of rhythmic modes, namely, briskness and heaviness; and the level of harmony and disposition that the different pulse beats reach is comparable to the level of harmony and disposition that rhythmic beats and the proportions of rhythmic modes reach. To grasp these relations is difficult; they will be sensed only by someone accustomed to the method of rhythm and the harmony of modes, and who also possesses a knowledge of the science of music.[42]

This attitude had ancient roots. Galen already observed that "Every pulse has rhythm," and he, too, declared grounding in music to be necessary to the pulse taker.[43] And in fact the accent on rhythm went back still further, to Herophilus and the very beginnings of pulse diagnosis.

Herophilus defined rhythm as the ratio of the duration of the artery's diastole to the duration of its systole, and he considered it a singularly revealing sign. Its changes mirrored a person's progression from infancy through adolescence, to maturity and old age. Each stage of life had a characteristic cadence:

The pulse of the neonate is very small, and one distinguishes neither the systole nor the diastole. Herophilus says that this pulse has no definite proportion (*alogon*).... The first pulse which one can discern in a child assumes the rhythm of a foot composed of short syllables; it is short in both the diastole and the systole, and one therefore recognizes the two-beat (*dichronos*; i.e., pyrrhic). Among those who are older, the pulse is similar to what they (the grammarians) call the *trochee*: it has three beats, of which the diastole takes up two and the systole one. In the pulse of adults, the diastole is equal to the systole; one compares it to what is called the *spondee*: the longest of the two-syllable feet, and is composed of four beats.... The pulse of those past their prime and approaching old age is composed of three beats. The systole is long and takes up double the diastole (i.e., the iamb).[44]

There is a congruence, in other words, between the syllables that we speak and the communicativeness of the pulse, the language of life. Both are articulated by iambs, spondees, and trochees. Both are essentially musical.

Critics accused Herophilus here of abandoning practical medicine for idle speculation — a charge occasionally leveled as well against later musical efforts.[45] But music and medicine were bound together in part through a theory of the soul. The inquiries of the Pythagoreans reputedly included the art of melotherapy.[46] For Plato, as Edward Lippman remarks, musical order was "simply another aspect of the imitation of virtue, just as the harmony of the tripartite soul is a fundamental aspect of virtue itself."[47] This was one reason why harmonious music could induce human harmony. Completely to grasp the connections between harmony, rhythm, numbers, and the body, Plato declares in the *Philebus*, is to reach perfection:

> But when you have learned what sounds are high and what low, and the number and the nature of the intervals and their limits or proportions, and the systems compounded out of them, which our fathers discovered and have been handed down to us under the name of harmonies; and the affections corresponding to them in the movements of the human body, which when measured by numbers ought, as they say, to be called rhythms and measures; and they tell us that the same principles should be applied to every one and many; — when, I say, you have learned all this, my dear friend, you are perfect; and you may be said to understand any other subject, when you have a similar grasp of it.[48]

Although Lippman's translation conveys Plato's enthusiasm for music and his sense of its broad significance, it obscures some critical nuances. What he renders, "the same principles should be applied to every one and many," Hackforth more appropriately translates, "this is always the right way to deal with the one-and-many problem."[49] The real subject of the passage is not music per se, but the philosophical perplexities surrounding the theory of Forms — the problem, specifically, of how single Forms relate to the multiplicity of phenomena. In these remarks on music Socrates is trying to clarify a prior observation about a gift of the gods, a gift transmitted in the saying that "All things ... that are ever said to be consist of a one and a many, and have in their nature a conjunction of limit and unlimitedness."[50]

The world at once displays both irreducible diversity and hints of latent elemental unities. For instance: the infinite variety of the sounds that emerge from the mouth and the singleness of the letters of the alphabet. It is after citing this example of speech that Socrates presents the above commentary on music.

What is music about? Again, Hackforth's translation clarifies what Lippman's leaves dark. Lippman's reading, "the movements of the human body" (*en tais kinēsesin tou sōmatos*), fails to tell us what these movements have to do with music. Comparison of this passage with discussions of music elsewhere in Plato, however, supports Hackforth's more explanatory gloss: "the performer's bodily movements." At issue is dance.

Plato frequently cites harmony and rhythm together. The former qualified the singing voice, the latter the movements of dance.[51] This reflects a prime feature of Greek music, and one that Lippman himself stresses, namely, that, "the combination of poetry, melody, and dance ... was the ideal type of music as well the predominant type."[52] Music encompassed not just melody and the theory of harmony, but also dance and verse, and the theory of rhythm.

But what is rhythm? A final contrast between the Lippman and Hackforth versions. Movements are characterized, in Lippman's translation, by "rhythms and measures." But Hackforth gives instead the startling rendering, "figures and measures." He translates *rhythmos* as "figure."

Rhythmos first appears in Greek literature among the early elegaic poets, where the word seems to mean something like "disposition."[53] By the fifth century, we find various authors using it in the sense of "shape" or "form." Thus Herodotus in referring to Hellenistic modifications of the Phoenician alphabet notes how the Greeks "changed the *rhythmos* of the letters,"[54] and the Atomists Democritus and Leucippus similarly identified *rhythmos* as one of the three causes of perceptible phenomena. Aristotle in his report of Atomist teachings elaborates: "Rhythm is form" (*rhythmos schēma estin*).[55]

It is against this background that we must read later writers such as Diodorus Siculus, who speaks of the "*rhythmos* of the ancient statues in Egypt," and Diogenes Laertius, who notes that Pythagoras, a sculptor from Rhegion, "seems to have been the first to aim at *rhythmos* and *symmetria*."[56] Before the fourth century B.C.E., the term seems to have been as important to the appreciation of sculpture as to the analysis of music.[57]

Yet if rhythm meant form, how did it become fused to motion and to music? Eugen Petersen's classic analysis of 1917 identified the crucial bridge in dance. Petersen's insight, J. J. Pollitt summarizes, was that

> *rhythmoi* were originally the "positions" that the human body was made to assume in the course of a dance, in other words the patterns or *schemata* that the body made. In the course of a dance certain obvious patterns or positions, like the raising or lowering of a foot, were naturally repeated, thus making intervals in the dance. Since

88

music and singing were synchronized with dancing, the recurrent positions taken by the dancer in the course of his movements also marked distinct intervals in the music; the rhythmoi of the dancer thus became the rhythmoi of the music. This explains why the basic component of music and poetry was called a *pous*, "foot" (Plato, *Rep.* 400a), or *basis*, "step" (Aristotle, *Metaph.* 1087b37) and why, within the foot, the basic elements were called the *arsis*, "lifting, up-step," and *thesis*, "placing, down-step."[58]

A dramatic performance presents a continuous stream of varying melodies, words, and gestures. *Rhythmoi* were the fixed patterns and positions of dance that endowed them all with visible articulate structure.

Werner Jaeger concludes similarly:

Rhythm, then, is that which imposes bonds on movement and confines the flux of things ... Obviously, when the Greeks speak of the rhythm of a building or a statue, it is not a metaphor transferred from musical language; the original conception that lies beneath the Greek discovery of rhythm in music and dancing is not *flow* but *pause*, the steady limitation of movement.[59]

Reflected in the idea of rhythm, in other words, was the impulse to seek (and literally see) the meaning of change in unchanging, definite forms. Jaeger's remarks support Hackforth's translation of *rhythmoi* and shed light on Socrates' use of rhythm in dance as an example of the one-and-the-many, that is, of "the conjunction of the limited and the unlimited."[60] In the same way that fixed, eternal Forms underlay the variety and ceaseless flux of the phenomenal world, so *rhythmoi*, signifying positions, ordered and limited the movements of dance.

And so it was that rhythm came to define as well the semantic skeleton of the pulse. Diastole and systole corresponded to arsis and thesis, the raising of the foot and the lowering of the foot. Herophilus, Galen reports,

> has written concerning the time intervals of systole and diastole, and reduced their proportions into rhythms varying in accordance with age. For just as musicians arrange the time lengths of notes comparing "rise" (*arsis*) and "fall" (*thesis*) with each other according to determinate time intervals, so also Herophilus, regarding "rise" as analogous to diastole and "fall" as analogous to systole, began his examination with the newborn child. He postulated a quasi-atomic minimum perceptible time unit, the interval occupied by the expansion of the infant's artery, and he also says that the systole or contraction is measured by an equal time unit, but he makes no clear definition of either of the periods of quiet.[61]

The final remark about periods of quiet bears special comment. In Galen's eyes, one flaw in Herophilus' theory of the pulse was the failure explicitly to recognize the pauses punctuating the transition from diastole to systole and, again, from systole to diastole.[62] The ratio of diastole to systole, Galen insisted, represented only part of the message contained in a single beat; no less significant was the ratio between the durations of each of these two motions and durations of the two rest periods that separated them.[63] Indeed, he regarded a true appreciation of these rests as one of the chief achievements of post-Herophilean sphygmology.

The musical theorist Aristoxenus held that "rhythm is composed of an alternation of movements and rests. The rests are the syllable, the note, or the position of a dance; movement is necessary to pass from one of these elements to another. These transitions are instantaneous."[64]

Pauses thus defined the very heart of the idea of rhythm. It was the still stance that signified; movements were mere transitions. Doctors interpreting the pulse allowed more meaning to motions, recognizing distinct and vital functions in the artery's diastole and systole. But Aristoxenus' comments help to clarify Galen's preoccupation with the rests between them — rests that mechanical sphygmographs would eventually expose as fictions. Just as the positions of pause articulated the meaning of dance, just as Myron's sculpture captured the essence of the whirling blur of an athlete hurling a discus in a dynamic revealing pose (figure 14), so the message of the artery's dilations and contractions could only be understood by reference to the rests that punctuated them.

Previous commentaries on the musical interpretation of the pulse have related it mostly to beliefs about the soul as a sort of harmony, and health as a kind of attunement.[65] But this neglects how the communication between music and pulse theory passed through rhythm rather than harmony, and it obscures the revealing hint contained in the original sense of rhythm as form.

Rhythm in pulse diagnosis merits study because the history of its analysis is long and rich, and stretches from antiquity to the modern electrocardiograph; merits study, too, because, as the ratio of diastole and systole — the balance between the artery's dilation and contraction — rhythm spotlights the very essence of the pulse. But I have lingered on it for another reason: the concept of rhythm reflects certain habits of mind. In the congruence between the *rhythmoi* of sculpture, music, and medicine we glimpse a recurring approach to interpretation, an insistence on seeking the meaning of expressive change — the message of speech, say, or the pulse, or dance — in elements that themselves don't change. Ideas and numbers. Still shapes.

Chinese doctors knew no equivalent to rhythm, and this most obviously because the *mo*, unlike the pulse, wasn't composed of a

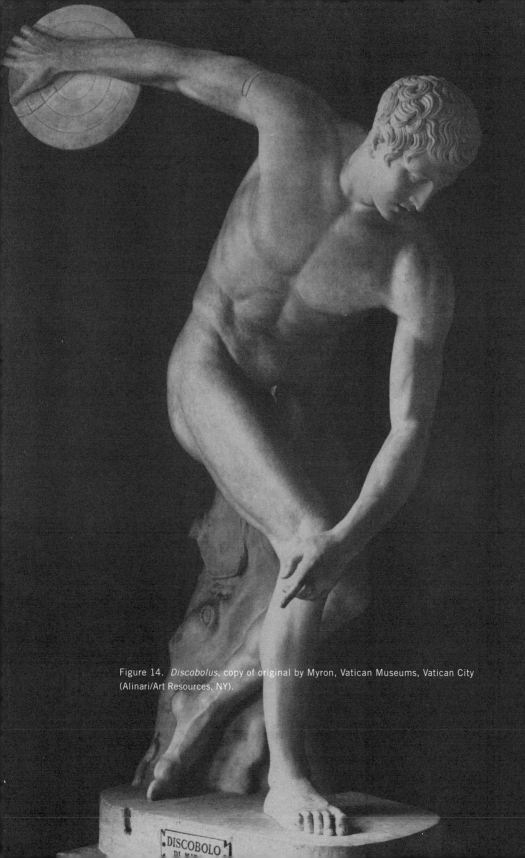

Figure 14. *Discobolus*, copy of original by Myron, Vatican Museums, Vatican City (Alinari/Art Resources, NY).

systole and a diastole. But this contrast in conceptions of the objects of interpretation, of the sources of meaning, may in turn be inseparable from a broader, more basic contrast — a difference in the very understanding of how things mean.

Ciqi, or the Spirit of Words

Wang Shuhe's *Mojing* sets forth straightaway, in the opening section of the very first volume, the core vocabulary of the language of the *mo* — a list of its twenty-four major variations.

Floating *mo*: if one lifts the fingers there is abundance; if one presses down one finds insufficiency

Hollow *mo*: floating, large and soft; pressing down the center is vacuous and the two sides feel full

Flooding *mo*: extremely large under the fingers

Slippery *mo*: it comes and goes in fluid succession; similar to the rapid

Rapid *mo*: it comes and goes with urgent haste

Intermittent *mo*: after coming and going several times, it stops once and then returns

Chordlike *mo*: if one lifts the fingers there is nothing; if one presses down it feels like a bowstring

Tense *mo*: like palpating a rope

Sunken *mo*: if one lifts the fingers it is lacking; pressing down one encounters abundance

Hidden *mo*: pressing down extremely hard, one finds the pulse when one reaches the bone

Leathery *mo*: as if sunken, hidden, full, large, and long with a hint of the chordlike

Full *mo*: large and long and slightly strong; when one presses down it hides beneath the fingers; firm

Faint *mo*: extremely thin and soft as if about to disappear; it appears both to be there and not to be there

93

Rough *mo*: thin and slow, coming and going with difficulty, dispersing; sometimes it will stop and then resume

Thin *mo*: small, but more prominent than faint; though thin, it persists

Soft *mo*: extremely soft and floating, thin

Weak *mo*: extremely soft, sunken, and thin; when one presses down it nearly disappears

Empty *mo*: slow, large and soft; pressing down one finds it lacking, and it hides under the fingers; vacuous

Dispersing *mo*: large and dispersing; this indicates excess *qi* and insufficient blood

Lazy *mo*: coming and going are like slow, but slightly faster than slow

Slow *mo*: the *mo* arrives only three times during one respiratory cycle; it comes and goes extremely slowly

Halting *mo*: it comes and goes lazily, stops, and then resumes

Faltering *mo*: it comes several times, then stops, and is scarcely able to resume

Moving *mo*: observed at the *guan* position, it has no head nor tail; it is about the size of a pea; it wavers, swaying[66]

Such was the world of palpation in China — a dense, tangled mesh of interrelated, interpenetrating sensations. A faint *mo* is "extremely soft and thin"; a weak *mo* is "extremely soft, sunken, and thin"; a thin *mo* is "small, but more prominent than faint"; a soft *mo* is "soft, floating, and thin." Qualities thus defined themselves and each other, clustering closely, and differing by fine, gossamer veils of sensation, subtle shades of faintness, weakness, softness. No trace here of crisp categories such as size, speed, rhythm, and frequency — the geometrical logic of space, time, and number. The rapid *mo* was a relative of the slippery, the rough mo resembled the halting.[67] In the porousness of the intercourse among words, we couldn't be further from the sharp de-

94

marcations that European doctors thought necessary to a secure science.

What expectations accompanied utterances like "floating," "hollow," "tense," "chordlike"? What kind of gesture was it when a doctor taught the disciple, "A flooding *mo* is extremely large under the fingers"? We can say: he was asserting a fact. But this isn't enough. "I have no money," also states a fact, but depending on the tone and circumstances, the statement may be a joke or an accusation, a plea for clemency or a pitch for a loan. Words have countless uses, and the same phrases can, in disparate contexts with altered intonations, instill fear or elicit laughter. The question remains: What sort of assertion was "A flooding *mo* is extremely large under the fingers"? How should we read traditional utterances on the *mo*?

We could suppose the master explaining, "The flooding *mo* is one that is extremely large under the fingers," in response to the query "What is a flooding *mo*?" Read thus, "Extremely large under the fingers" resembles a definition, a statement of fact. Except for one peculiarity: the definition identifies the flooding *mo* by specifying its relationship to the fingers. It asserts what the flooding *is* by describing how it *feels*.

Greek pulse theory, we learned above, sought strictly to segregate what a pulse is from how it feels, fact from perception. In the tetralogy that formed the core of his sphygmological writings, Galen devoted the first treatise, *Peri diaphoras sphygmōn* (On differences between pulses), to expounding the defining characteristics of each pulse in and of itself, objectively, independent of the touching of it. He then outlined how to distinguish these pulses, perceptually, in a second and separate work, *Peri diagnōseōs sphygmōn* (On the discernment of pulses).

By contrast, in Wang Shuhe's glosses on such *mo* as the floating and the sunken, the hollow and the hidden, the full and the weak, the question of the identity of a *mo* blends indistinguishably into the issues of haptic technique. Place your fingers lightly and the *mo* is there; press down and the *mo* disappears. That is how one knows the floating *mo*. Place your fingers lightly and you find nothing; press down and the *mo* appears. Such is the sunken *mo*. A *mo* feels floating, large and soft, but when the fingers push in, they encounter an emptiness in the center while the two sides feel full. So you recognize a hollow *mo*. Each *mo* responds differently to the inquiring hand, and it is by their differing responses that one tells them apart.

"If one lifts the fingers there is abundance; if one presses down one finds insufficiency." To us, this reads like a reply to "How does one grasp a floating *mo*?" rather than to the question "What is a floating *mo*?" But in China the manner in which a *mo* was experienced was integral to its essence. To know the floating or the sunken, the hollow or the hidden, the full or the weak was to know how they appeared to the probing touch. Asking "what" was inseparable from asking "how."

The attitude wasn't unique to medicine. Listen to these exchanges about filial piety in the *Analects*:

> Meng Yizi asked about (*wen*) filial piety. Confucius said: "Never disobey." [Later,] when Fan Chi was driving him, Confucius told him, "Mengsun asked me about filial piety, and I answered him, 'Never disobey.'" Fan Chi said, "What does that mean?" Confucius said, "When parents are alive, serve them according to the rules of propriety. When they die, bury them according to the rules of propriety and sacrifice to them according to the rules of propriety."
>
> Meng Wubo asked about filial piety. Confucius said, "Especially be anxious lest parents should be sick."
>
> Ziyu asked about filial piety. Confucius said, "Filial piety nowadays means to be able to support one's parents. But we support even

dogs and horses. If there is no feeling of reverence, wherein lies the difference?"[68]

Wing-tsit Chan here renders the Chinese verb *wen* as "ask about." The translation is perfectly appropriate, yet as English usage it is faintly odd. We ask about our friend's health, we ask about the possibility of rain, but we don't usually ask *about* concepts. Or when we do, we have some more specific question in mind, like "How does filial piety square with public responsibility?" or "What do you think of John's interpretation of filial piety?" or simply, "What does filial piety mean?"

Confucius's replies suggest that none of these queries really corresponds to *wen*. Again, as with the characterizations of the various *mo*, we are almost tempted to read here an inquiry about method — something like, "How does one become filial?" When Fan Chi follows up on the Master's answer of "Never disobey" and voices the Socratic-sounding challenge "What does that mean?," Confucius merely tenders more instructions about proper filial conduct. Serve your parents with reverence. Don't let them get sick. Bury them properly. As if to *wen* filial piety was to ask simultaneously "What is filial piety?" and "How does one become filial?"

Now one reason for Confucius's changing answers may lie in the maxim that individuals should be taught according to their abilities. But the variety of his responses to the same query almost certainly reflects as well the assumption that learning words is like learning all skills — it involves mastering an indefinite range of attitudes and patterns of behavior. If we ask about archery, for instance, the instructor might initially advise, "Keep your eyes on the target" and suggest at another time, "The secret is to hold the head level." On still another occasion we might be told, "Archery is the art of perfect relaxation." Yet none of these instructions, singly or together, exhausts the art of archery. A real archer must know all these things and more.

Grasping the *mo* was similar. Disciples of Wang Shuhe couldn't ask "What is a floating pulse?" in the same way that young Greek doctors challenged Galen to state fixed discrete definitions. For Chinese terms didn't refer to objective states of the artery — the diameter of its expansion, say, or the speed of its contraction. Learning about the floating *mo* was more like learning about filial piety. This is why, instead of being doubted and debated, the vocabulary of the *mo* was continually redescribed — in similes, in metaphors, in that imaginative style that later European doctors found so extravagant.

Wang Shuhe said of the floating *mo*: "If one lifts the fingers there is abundance, if one presses down one finds insufficiency." Physicians after him proffered other, more vivid characterizations. "Like clouds floating in the sky," Li Gao suggested. "Buoyant, like wood floating on water," explained Li Zhongzi. "The floating *mo*," Li Shizhen elaborated expansively, "is like a subtle breeze blowing across the down of a bird's back. It is quiet and whispering, like falling elm pods, like wood floating in water, like scallion leaves rolled lightly between the fingers."[69]

This style went back to the ancient classics. "The normal *mo* for the lungs is quiet and whispering like falling elm pods," the *Suwen* relates; when the lungs falter, the *mo* feels "suspended, and one has a sensation of stroking a rooster feather." As they fail and death nears, the *mo* recalls "feathers blown by the wind." A healthy liver *mo* "comes soft weak and quivering, like the tip of a long pole," but when the liver is afflicted, the *mo* feels "full, firm, slippery, like a long pole." When the sickness turns fatal, the *mo* "is tense and taut, like a freshly strung bowstring."[70]

Nothing could have been more alien to the Galenic ideal of literalness. Here was language that conjured up metaphorical simulacra rather than speaking directly of the arteries, their states and movements; here were descriptions that focused exclusively on how the pulse might appear to the perceiver, and revealed nothing about the underlying realities. As if the *mo* lacked concrete palpable presence.

Graphic representations of the *mo* displayed a similar indirectness. A baffled John Floyer remarked: "Chinese pictures of the pulse are pure hieroglyphics, and not yet explained to us." Floyer felt that these pictures, just like Chinese representations of the viscera and of men and women more generally, lacked "exactness; a little similitude they think sufficient."[71] The illustrations in Shi Fa's *Chabing zhinan* typify how the *mo* was portrayed in traditional China (figure 13). Do the large rings here depict blood vessels? Perhaps, or perhaps not, it scarcely matters. They betray no trace of motion, are identical in size, and contribute nothing to distinguishing one *mo* from another. The meaning of each representation lay entirely in the patterns inscribed within.

How were readers supposed to interpret these bubbles and dots, lines and squiggles? Shi Fa doesn't say. But it is plain that these pictures weren't intended to be read like blueprints, in which each mark maps a discrete detail; it is plain that the message of each sketch lay instead in the overall impression, the total effect. Other treatises evoked the same *mo* with other designs (figures 15, 16, 17). Understanding a *mo* entailed seeing what it was *like*. There was nothing more exact, more basic, more real to be known.

Chapter 1 taught us that the *mo* were visible in the bulging blood vessels of frightened horses and could be seen in humans emerging and entering near the surface of the body, at the joints. We shall discover in later chapters that Chinese healers actually drew blood from the *mo*, and that Han dynasty dissectors even inserted bamboo strips into them to trace their courses and mea-

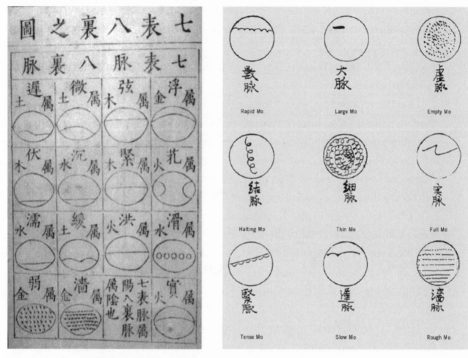

Figure 15. *Mojue*, Shanghai Medical University.
Figure 16. Saka Jōun, *Zoku tenkō hōhi yōshō*, Fujikawa Collection, Kyoto University Library.

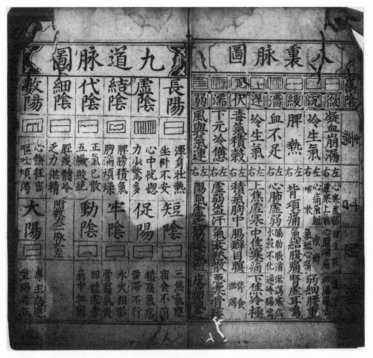

Figure 17. *Mojing conghuang*, Shanghai Library.

sure their lengths. The *mo*, in other words, didn't always or necessarily lack concrete presence. But when they were palpated by doctors seeking to know the past, present, and future of their patients, they were handled quite differently than when they were measured in dissection or cut to release blood. Doctors deployed a separate touch in *qiemo*, for there they were interested not in distances or pathways or sites of surgical intervention, but in something else.

> When *qi* and blood are strong, then the *mo* is strong; when the *qi* and blood decline, then the *mo* declines. When the *qi* and blood are hot then the *mo* is rapid; when the *qi* and blood are chilled, then the *mo* is slow. When the *qi* and blood are feeble, then the *mo* is weak. When the *qi* and blood are calm, then the *mo* is relaxed.[72]

Qiemo was palpation of the *mo*, but this *mo*, in Hua Tuo's (141–208) classic formula, was "the manifestation of *qi* and blood" (*mo zhe, qixue zhi xian ye*). Doctors prized the *mo* because of its exquisite sensitivity (the term *xian*, "manifestation," carried implications of what is first, prior, incipient) to changes in blood and *qi*. Or sometimes, simply *qi*. Explained the *Suwen*:

> When the *mo* is long, then the *qi* is settled. When the *mo* is short, then the *qi* is ailing. When the *mo* is rapid, the heart is troubled. When the *mo* is large, then the ailment is progressing. When the upper part of the *mo* rules, then the *qi* has risen. When its lower part rules, then the *qi* is swollen. When the *mo* is intermittent, then the *qi* is weak. When the *mo* is thin, then *qi* is lacking.[73]

What was at stake in such changes? Why was it important to know when *qi* became chilled or heated, or weak, or calm, when it rose, and when it swelled? The passage from Hua Tuo continues, revealingly: "A tall person has a long *mo*; a short person has a short *mo*. [A person with] a tense nature has a tense *mo*; [a person with] a relaxed nature has a relaxed *mo*." It wasn't just blood and *qi* that were manifest in the *mo*, but people's very natures. That is to say: to know blood and *qi* was to know the person.

The earliest references to *qi* and *xueqi* (blood and *qi*) appear in the *Analects*. "The person of superior cultivation guards against three things," the Master cautions: "When he is young and the blood and qi are not yet settled, he guards against lust. When he matures, and the blood and qi are in full vigor, he guards against combativeness. When he is old, and the blood and qi have declined, he guards against covetousness."[74]

Blood and *qi* were thus associated from the beginning with core aspects of a person's being. Confucius conceived them as obscure tides of raw, latent powers pulling darkly, fiercely against the resolution toward virtue. Changes in blood and *qi* ruled the transitions between lust, aggression, and greed.

We can read Confucius's warnings anachronistically as a sort of crude psychophysiology, as primitive insights into the terrifying influence of hormones — if we bear in mind that blood and *qi* were known otherwise than by chemical analysis, that the heart of their reality lay in personal experience. When doctors in the *Neijing* subsequently spoke of *qi* rising in anger, sinking in fear, seeping away in sorrow, they weren't so much trying to *explain* emotions, objectively, as relating what they knew from their own bodies, describing what they felt, subjectively, within themselves. In anger, a sudden, explosive surge; in grief, a draining away. It was the intimate everyday familiarity of such sensations that made the traditional discourse of vital flux so compelling. The deepest certainties about *qi* were rooted in knowledge that people had of the body because they *were*, themselves, bodies.[75]

At the same time, however — and this point merits emphasis —

the experience of *qi* was never purely internal. *Qi* was subjectively felt, but it was also perceptible from without. Doctors eventually seized it with their fingers, palpating its ebb and flow in the *mo*. And before that Confucius already drew attention to the interplay between who a person was and how a person spoke — between self and language. "There are three things that the person of superior cultivation values most in the Way," the Master said; one of them is "to avoid being vulgar and contrary by speaking in proper tones (*ciqi*)."[76] It was especially in the *ciqi* — the *qi* of words — that he heard a person's deeper commitments.

The Confucian thinker Mencius (371–289 B.C.E.) vaunted two special talents. One was an aptitude for cultivating his "floodlike *qi*," a vitality nourished by moral discipline; the other was a knack for knowing words (*zhi yan*). Coming from a philosopher, the latter boast might lead us to suppose a talent for analyzing terms. But Mencius actually referred to a different sort of skill: "When words are extravagant, I know how the mind is fallen and sunk. When words are depraved, I know how the mind has departed from principle. When words are evasive, I know how the mind is at its wit's end."[77]

Knowing words thus meant understanding what words reveal about those who speak them — hearing the attitudes and dispositions from which they spring. Just as we would be wrong to seek the meaning of individual bubbles and squiggles in Shi Fa's depictions of the *mo*, so Mencius didn't interpret words singly, as symbols for discrete ideas. He listened instead to the broad flow of discourse, its drift, and knew that here was a feckless schemer and there a man gripped by desperation.

Of course, in many circumstances we too listen in this way. We know that what a person is saying may have nothing to do, really, with what he or she seems to be talking about — the change in the weather, the price of eggs. We can hear the desire for reconciliation, or the deliberate intent to hurt. Indeed, many of our quarrels arise precisely because, sometimes, we can't help but listen in this way. "What's that supposed to mean?" someone snaps, querulous and suspicious, hearing insult veiled in idle chatter. An angry mother who exclaims, "Don't take that tone with me!" knows that her son's "Yes, mother," voices more sullen resistance than docile assent. Anyone can mouth the required phrases. But their real significance — as judged by how listeners react, by whether they are offended, or moved, or mollified — often turns on how the phrases are uttered.

How we hear cruelty or kindness or pompous pretense can seem a mystery. For at times, we are quite deaf. "You aren't listening!" complains an exasperated friend. Perhaps we are preoccupied, or biased toward what we want to hear. Certainly we differ in acuity. Some, like Mencius presumably, can discern even inclinations unacknowledged by the speakers themselves; others listening to the same words hear nothing. Moreover, even when we do hear we are often unable to say what exactly we are hearing, whether it is the diction, or inflection, or pitch that clues us in. The most revealing words, taken one by one and without context, are often perfectly ordinary.

Yet the matter may be plain enough. Perhaps we hear fear or kindness as directly as we hear a cat's meowing, or someone whistling in the dark. The mystery may be an artifact of supposing that we *really* hear something else — individual words, say, and convert them through some arcane, but lightning-quick hermeneutic into inferences about inner states — when, experientially, we have no sense of interpreting. Someone says angry words, and we hear angry words.

Of course, we don't *always* hear in this manner. In some contexts, as in lending an ear to a public announcement, we are scarcely aware of the speaker and attend only to the information. Or again, certain kinds of philosophizing invite us to meditate on isolated terms in the abstract, as impersonal counters for ideas. We listen in different ways because language is used in different ways.

Styles of speaking are shaped partly by what is being spoken of. Once we recognize the disparate natures of the objects that they handled, we can understand why the vocabularies of pulse taking and *qiemo* should differ so: the relevant distinctions naturally wouldn't be the same for analyzing the pulsing artery, and for describing streams of blood and *qi*. There is a world of difference between calculating rhythm and palpating for slipperiness and roughness.

That the *uses* of words should diverge, too, makes sense. Writers on the pulse demanded lucid and direct descriptions, free of metaphorical shadows, not least because they identified the pulse with the clear crisp image of the tubular artery, because they conceived it as an idea, something seen, a geometric form envisioned in the mind's eye. Whereas the *mo* flowed and lacked sharp contours.

Sometimes the *mo* coursed smoothly, at other times it was rough; sometimes it floated along the surface, dispersing at the slightest pressure, at other times, one had to press down deep to engage its currents. Definitions could scarcely be more precise than the bare names for these *mo*: slippery, rough, floating, sunken. Graphically, such fluid qualities could be pictured only indirectly, by suggestion, by undulating lines and arching bubbles. Verbally, clarifications of the floating *mo* could do no more than evoke billowing clouds in the sky, the dreamy descent of elm seeds, the down on a bird's back blowing in the light breeze.

Yet in the end, the problem of how people speak goes deeper than the question of what they are speaking about. Yes, styles of speaking about the *mo* and the pulse differed radically, *in part* because the *mo* and the pulse were radically disparate realities. But the preceding remarks on Mencian knowledge of words, and before that the discussions of the pulse taker's quest for literalism, remind us that styles of speaking are also inseparable from styles of listening. We speak in a certain manner expecting to be heard in a certain manner; and conversely, the way in which we listen to others depends on our assumptions about how they are expressing meaning and, indeed, our conceptions of what meaning is.

What makes such interdependence especially significant for a history of haptic knowledge is this: if speaking and listening were tightly intertwined, so in turn were listening and touching. Just as Confucius and Mencius attended closely to the *qi* of words, so in medical diagnosis doctors sought out the fluctuations of *qi* in the *mo*. If the *mo* was the manifestation of blood and *qi*, "Blood and *qi*," Hua Shou specified, constitute a "person's *shen*."[78] In everyday language *shen* referred most often to gods and divinities, but in medicine the term gestured toward the ineffable yet palpable difference between a stony cadaver and a breathing, responsive human being — the spirit of a person, the divine essence of life. *Qiemo*, in other words, entailed touching a person in a manner parallel to the way we listen when a friend says, "I don't care anymore," but we hear in her tone the bitter lingering regret; when we listen, that is, not for the abstract impersonal meaning of single words, but hear the latent spirit behind them.

Restated more generally, my thesis is that the history of conceptions of the body must be understood in conjunction with a history of conceptions of communication. When Greek and Chinese doctors palpated the body, they were guided not only by specific beliefs about the arteries and the *mo* and the organization of the body, but also by broader assumptions about the nature of human expressiveness. In seeking to understand people doctors in each tradition often felt with their fingers in much the same way that they listened with their ears.

The arts of pulse diagnosis and *qiemo* arose from the conviction that people express themselves not just in words, in a language accessible to the ears, but also in a language accessible only to the touch. Sometimes, as in the Greek assimilation of the syllables of speech with the rhythmical articulations of the pulse, doctors drew explicit parallels between these two forms of expression. More often, though, they simply took it for granted that the style in which the body communicated messages by palpable movements would resemble how people conveyed meaning by the voice.

PART TWO

Styles of Seeing

CHAPTER THREE

Muscularity and Identity

"Why can't you see?"

Shouted in the course of an argument, the plaint often voices genuine bewilderment mixed with anger. Bewilderment, because to the speaker the matter seems as clear as day. How could any-one not see? Anger, because given the obviousness of the matter, the failure to see kindles suspicions of willful obtuseness, per-verse prejudice. Though we may allow abstractly for the relativ-ity of perspectives, our own viewpoint is often so vivid that it doesn't seem like a viewpoint at all, but simply the way things are.

It is a powerful optical illusion.

Comparing the musculature portrayed in Vesalius' anatomy and the total absence of muscles in the acupuncture man, we see almost irresistibly a puzzle about blindness, about how observant Chinese doctors overlooked, strangely, one of the most promi-nent features of the human body. Yet historically, the vision of muscularity was in fact the exception. Interest in individual mus-cles and indeed the very notion of muscles — as distinct from flesh, tendons, and sinews — developed uniquely in medical traditions rooted in ancient Greece. Elsewhere, as in China, "ignorance" of musculature was the rule.

So the real puzzle concerns sight not blindness. It makes little sense to wonder why the Chinese failed to observe muscles when such failure was the norm. Of course, we can and should explore the question of what doctors in China *did* see; but that is the task of chapter 4. My focus here is the enigma of the European muscular body — the problem of the peculiar vantage point from which muscles came to look natural and self-evident and impossible to miss.

Chapters 1 and 2 delved into how gestures could appear the same yet differ radically in the experience; they probed alternative styles of touching. This chapter and the next elucidate alternative ways of seeing.

Muscularity and Art

Present intuitions about human muscularity owe much to the history of Western art. We are startled by Chinese "neglect" of musculature in no small part because an influential tradition of representing the body, stretching from the fifth century B.C.E. and the metopes of the Parthenon (figure 18) through the "ten naked men" of Antonio Pollaiuolo (1432–98) (figure 19) and beyond, has accustomed us to imagining muscles as salient perspicuous structures that we have merely to look to see.

In fact, this is an illusion — as a survey of any summer beach reveals: most muscles on most people in most circumstances can be apprehended but obscurely, if at all. In his textbook on drawing of 1755, Charles-Antoine Jombert asseverated, "A beginner sees almost no muscles in a nude body." Envisioning musculature is an acquired skill.

To see as an artist must see, Jombert taught, students must learn anatomy — "to enable you to discover the whereabouts of the bones and muscles."[1] The trained gaze sees what the beginner's vague sight does not, because the anatomical eye knows exactly what it is supposed to perceive. It is a lesson that we must

112

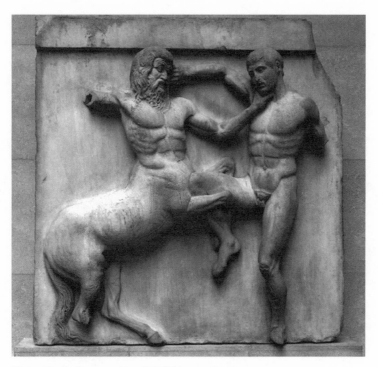

Figure 18. Parthenon metope, British Museum, London.

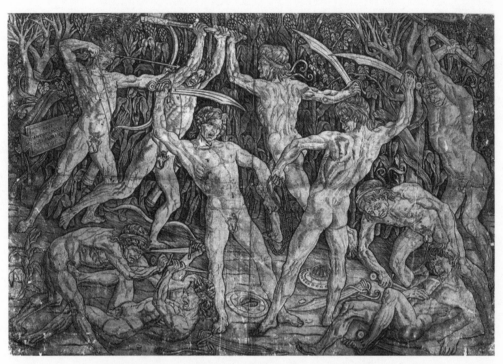

Figure 19. Antonio Pollaiuolo, *The Battle of the Ten Naked Men*, Metropolitan Museum of Art, Purchase, Joseph Pulitzer Bequest, 1917 (17.50.99), New York.

always bear in mind: the musculature so crisply delineated in engravings, paintings, and sculptures mirrored a vision of the body in which what was seen from the outside was inseparable from what was imagined, anatomically, beneath the skin and obscuring fat.

There was thus the constant danger of slipping from seeing toward projecting. Leonardo da Vinci may have been complaining of figures like Pollaiuolo's musclemen when he stressed that a painter must understand *which* muscles work in a given action, "and must emphasize the bulging of those muscles only, and not of the rest, as some painters do who think that they are showing off their draftsmanship when they draw nudes that are knotty and graceless — mere sacks of nuts."[2]

Jombert, too, felt bound to warn his students against the common crude mistake of drawing even "the muscles that you cannot see in the model just because you know they must be there."[3] Although he still stressed: without this knowledge one sees nothing.

In the end, it remained murky how much, and even whether, one could sift out the anatomy lessons in the memory from what one actually saw in the model. A student certainly went astray when these lessons made the model superfluous; yet it was equally certain that in these lessons lay the secret of artful seeing and convincing representation.

Alberti's recommendations on this point are memorable:

> To get the right proportions in painting living creatures, first visualize their bony insides, for bones, being rigid, establish fixed measurements. Then attach tendons and muscles in their places and finally clothe the bones and muscles with flesh and skin. You may object that... a painter has no concern with what he cannot see. So be it, but if to paint dressed figures you must first draw them nude and then dress them, so to paint nudes you must first situate the

bones and muscles before you cover them with flesh and skin in order to show clearly where the muscles are.[4]

In portraying the body, then, artists had always to keep in mind what lay beneath the smooth contours of the surface and "show clearly where the muscles are." Even where separate muscles could barely be distinguished, one had to remain intensely aware of their presence.

Why? The illusion that muscles leap out naturally and inevitably to the eye, I said, owes much to the exaggerated clarity of musculature in paintings and sculptures. But what motivated this exaggeration? Why were artists so intent on displaying muscularity?

The short answer is that they saw muscles as somehow essential to human identity. A body without the muscles, to paraphrase Alberti, was like clothes without the person. But this answer only leads to the further question: in what way were they essential? What made imagining muscles necessary to imagining the body?

Dissection must have something to do with the matter. Leonardo, Alberti, and Jombert all tell us explicitly: to perceive muscles on the living person, one must first study the anatomy of the dead. And this presumably is a significant reason why Chinese doctors didn't notice them — because in their perspective on the body dissection played only a minor role. To solve the enigma of the Western preoccupation with muscles, therefore, we must factor in the contributions of anatomical seeing.

But anatomical seeing is itself a mystery.

The Puzzle of Anatomical Seeing
Extensive evidence of systematic dissection first appears in the 4th century B.C.E., with Aristotle's studies of animals.[5] Around the same time, Diocles of Carystos is said to have written the first

treatise on anatomy, again of animals, though this work is lost.[6] Most historians of medicine, however, have skipped quickly over these investigations. Ludwig Edelstein's classic study of the history of anatomy in antiquity defined what has remained the prevailing problematic: "[D]issections and vivisections can be performed on animals; and on animals they were performed before the Alexandrian period. Why are they suddenly carried out on human beings in Alexandria? This is the decisive question in the history of anatomy."[7] For most historians, the "decisive question" about anatomy has revolved around Herophilus, Erasistratus, and the shift in Alexandrian times from animal to human dissection.[8]

Now the problem of the context that allowed investigators to study the human body with methods practiced before only on animals certainly merits analysis.[9] But this question of application presupposes the prior existence of a method, and more importantly, a desire. The various philosophical, religious, and cultural factors that scholars have hitherto identified as obstructing or permitting human dissection gain meaning only within the frame of a preexisting anatomical urge.

From a comparative perspective, it is especially this urge that intrigues. For fathoming the contrast between the Vesalian muscleman and Hua Shou's nonanatomical map of acupuncture tracts the pressing issue is not why human dissection became possible in Alexandria, but rather why earlier investigators like Aristotle and Diocles were already so keen to peer into animals — why dissection of *any* sort seemed meaningful and compelling.

Anatomy eventually became so basic to the Western conception of the body that it assumed an aura of inevitability. This is why historians have concentrated so much on the obstacles to its development — as if without these impediments the desire to know would translate necessarily into the desire to dissect, as if the willingness and the curiosity to observe were the same as the willingness and curiosity to anatomize. When we speak today of the body in the context of medicine we picture almost reflexively the muscles, nerves, blood vessels, and other organs revealed by the dissector's knife and dazzlingly displayed in atlases.

Historically, however, anatomy is an anomaly. Major medical traditions such as the Egyptian, Ayurvedic, and Chinese all flourished for thousands of years without privileging the inspection of corpses. For that matter even the treatises of Hippocrates, the reputed source of Western medical wisdom, manifest scarce interest in anatomical inquiry.[10]

And why should we expect otherwise? There are innumerable ways to know the body. The body can be investigated, for instance, by observing how it is affected by particular foods in particular circumstances. It can be apprehended, too, as something shaped by the environment, varying under the influence of airs, and waters, and places. There is also the detailed practical understanding that comes from studying how the body changes when it is burned, or bled, or needled in diverse ways, at disparate sites. Nor can we ignore the self-awareness gained through exercises that transform the self — through yogic meditation and breathing, say, or bodybuilding. All these methods yield abundant real insights. No natural bias requires seeking the truth of the body in the dismembered corpse.

So how did anatomy acquire its special authority? The question is crucial not only for explicating the muscular body, but also for thinking through, more generally, the disparity between figures 1 and 2. For the most salient difference in the perspectives of the two pictures is surely this: that one is anatomical while the other is not. Yet no sooner do we query anatomy's authority, than we confront a second, subtler, and logically prior problem, namely, What *is* anatomy?

Erwin Ackerknecht notes in his *Short History of Medicine* that,

118

"even in those primitive tribes which perform autopsies — they open bodies regularly in order to detect 'witchcraft principles' — anatomical knowledge is as poor as among those who perform no such autopsies."[11] Again, in discussing Aztec medicine, he muses, "[I]t is remarkable that there is no evidence of any high grade of anatomical knowledge in ancient Mexico, in spite of the fact that human sacrifice offered rich opportunities for observing human anatomy."[12]

For that matter, the Greeks themselves practiced extispication, or divination by entrails.[13] Plato's notion of the liver as the mirror of the mind offers an evocative reminder of the haruspical practices that attained such sophistication among the Babylonians and Etruscans, and which these peoples presumably passed on to the Greeks.[14] Unknown in Homeric times, the examination of entrails entered official Greek religion around the time of Solon, supplanting the authority of ornithomancy. In Cyprus, Zeus was honored as "the dissector of entrails";[15] and throughout Greek history leaders and diviners queried the innards of sacrificed animals before embarking on wars and expeditions.[16]

Belief in truths hidden within bodies was thus widespread in antiquity, and to the casual observer, the actions of the hieroscopic soothsayer and the post-Hippocratic anatomist may have looked the same. But they weren't the same. Whatever the resemblance in gestures, extispication and medical dissection represented very different sorts of endeavors.[17] Which is to say: there must be more to anatomy than curiosity about secrets inscribed in the body and a willingness to use the knife.

What set apart the vision of the dissector from the diviner's gaze?[18] Although many ancient cultures (including the Chinese, as we shall later learn) cut open and scrutinized the interior of animals and humans, they didn't all look in the same manner, nor see the same things.[19] The fundamental puzzle of anatomy concerns

119

the crystallization of a particular way of peering into the body, the birth of a certain visual style.

The Babylonians regularly probed inside animals, for instance, and the models they constructed of the liver show that they boasted a sharp eye. Yet they developed nothing like the Greek understanding of somatic structure. Why? They possessed both the opportunity and the skill. Henry Sigerist hypothesized that what they lacked was the motivation: "A people that was able to represent the finest movements of the animal, that was accustomed to observe the smallest variations of the animal liver, would have been able to unveil the secrets of the organism to a certain degree — *if it had felt the urge to do so*" (italics added).[20]

Anatomy involves a distinct urge, a special desire. So perhaps the divergence in ways of seeing derived from a difference in objectives. Perhaps diviners saw entrails as signs of a more significant reality, perhaps they sought to see the past and the future, whereas anatomists eyed the body *as* the body — their aim was to know the body itself. Yet what could it mean, really, to distinguish between looking at something as a sign and seeing it as itself? How many kinds of looking are there? Ackerknecht says of dissection: "[T]he mere technique means nothing for scientific knowledge as long as it is not pervaded by the scientific spirit. With this spirit the opening of the bodies is an inexhaustible source of knowledge."[21] But by itself this explains nothing. Precisely at issue is the character of a gaze pervaded by "the scientific spirit" — the nature of anatomical seeing.

It is a famous feature of classical Greek that a great number of words relating to cognition appeal to the experience of sight. Explicating the Homeric concept of *noos*, for example, Bruno Snell remarks that the verbal form *noein* means "to acquire a clear mental image of something. Hence the significance of *noos*. It is the mind as the recipient of clear images, or more briefly, the organ of clear images.... *Noos* is, as it were, the mental eye which exercises an unclouded vision."[22]

Aeschylus speaks likewise of "an understanding endowed with eyes" (*phrena ōmmatōmenēn*), and Pindar of a "blind heart" (*tuphlon ētor*).[23] And from the verb *ideō*, "I see," derive the nouns *idea* and *eidos* — form, image, sort, and in Plato's philosophy, the sole objects of *epistēmē*, true science.[24] The haunting myth of the cave plays on just this elision of seeing and knowing.[25]

In this sense, we may find it natural that a cultural tradition so primed to the eye should nurture anatomy, a science so devoted to observation. But such generalities hardly constitute an explanation. It is one thing to muse poetically or philosophically about sight and insight; the messy inspection of entrails is something else. A vast chasm separates Plato's luminous vision of the Good from the gutting of bloody cadavers. The problem remains: Why and how did dissectors look?

Today the motivation that springs immediately to mind is that dissection is medically useful, even necessary. We thus are easily swayed by the Dogmatist argument, reported by Celsus, that "Since pains and various kinds of diseases arise in the interior parts...no one can apply remedies for them who is ignorant of the parts themselves. Therefore, it is necessary to cut into the bodies of the dead, and examine their viscera and intestines."[26]

But in antiquity this reasoning probably seemed less compelling. Ancient remedies, remember, didn't encompass the extensive surgical options made possible by modern anesthesia and antisepsis. Bleeding, exercise, massage, and above all the management of food and drugs — these were the chief cures available to the Greek doctor, and it is unclear how much their deployment would have been enhanced by the inspection of "viscera and intestines." A major stream of Greek doctors, indeed, dismissed anatomy on just these grounds. Thorough studies of symptoms and close observation of how various cures altered these symptoms — these and these alone, Empiricist doctors asserted, were the healer's concern.[27] Gazing upon entrails had no practical use.

Another point weighing against therapeutic application as a major motive for dissection is the fact that anatomical inquiry began not with humans, but with animals. Yes, to some extent, we might attribute this concentration on animals to the religious taboos surrounding the handling of the human corpse. Thus, in the time of the Roman Emperor Trajan, Rufus of Ephesus would ruefully reminisce, "We shall try to teach you how to name the internal parts by dissecting an animal that most closely resembles man.... In the past they used to teach this, more correctly, upon man."[28] Here the dissector turned to animals *faute de mieux*, as substitutes.

Such substitution, however, didn't always or necessarily imply an ulterior medical motive. Aristotle too remarks that "the inner parts of man are to a very great extent unknown" and urges the consequent need to examine the inner parts of animals similar to humans;[29] but nothing suggests that his pioneering investigations into anatomy were inspired or driven by the desire to relieve human suffering. His studies on animal structure and generation and habits make plain his desire to understand the logic governing all animals, and not just humans.

Even later, even when interest centered explicitly on human structure, therapeutic utility wasn't necessarily the sole or even chief concern. Galen complains, revealingly, that contemporary anatomists have "obviously elaborated with care the part of anatomy that is completely useless to physicians, or which gives little or only occasional help."[30] And he continues: "The most useful part of the science of anatomy lies in just that exact study neglected by professed experts. It would have been better to be ignorant of how many valves there are in each orifice of the heart, or how many vessels minister to it, or how or whence they come, or how the paired cranial nerves reach the brain, than not to know what muscles extend or flex the upper and lower arm and wrist, or thigh, leg, and foot."[31]

Both in scope and in detail, ancient anatomy extended far beyond the needs of ancient healers.

What motivated ancient dissectors, then? What did they seek to see? Besides doctors, Galen identifies three other sorts of anatomists: the naturalist (*anēr physikos*) who loves knowledge for its own sake; the individual who seeks only to show that Nature does nothing in vain; and the student of physical and mental functions.[32] Those familiar with Galen's *On the Usefulness of the Parts* will know that these three enterprises were often alternate faces of a single endeavor. To know the body was to see how Nature shaped each part perfectly for its end, that is to say, its use.

On the Usefulness of the Parts constitutes the most complete and detailed account of anatomical structure in antiquity. It is also, and not coincidentally, an epic meditation on the awe inspired by the body's divine design. With painstaking thoroughness Galen reviews how every feature of the body, however seemingly insignificant, is absolutely necessary, and displays Nature's foresight, and proves that "everything is so well-disposed that it couldn't possibly be better otherwise." When he inadvertently omits to contemplate the perfection manifest in the geometry of the optic nerves, he finds himself upbraided in a dream for "sinning against the Creator."[33] This is the tradition that Vesalius would later echo in his *Fabrica*, when he envisaged the body as the Great Creator's wisdom made manifest.[34] The core of anatomical curiosity lay here, in the vision of bodily forms as expressions of creative purpose.

Curiosity about final ends already framed the researches of Diocles of Carystos, whom Galen credits with the first treatise on anatomy. Erasistratus, the great Alexandrian anatomist, also stressed the "foresightful" (*pronoētikēn*) and "craftsmanlike" (*techniken*) character of Nature. Given the tradition that makes him a disciple of Aristotle's colleague Theophrastus, this doesn't surprise. Aristotle, in whom we find the first sure evidence of animal dissections, was also the most forceful and influential exponent of teleological analysis.[35]

Similarly, the one notable exception to the Hippocratic neglect of dissection, the treatise *On the Heart*, explicitly urged the contemplation of this organ as the product of crafty design:

> Close by the origin of the blood vessels certain soft and cavernous [or "porous"] bodies enfold the heart. Although they are called "ears" they are not perforated as ears are, nor do they hear any sound. They are in fact the instruments by which nature catches the air — the creation, as I believe, of an excellent craftsman, who seeing the heart would be a solid thing owing to the density of its material, and in consequence would have no attractive power, he equipped it with bellows, as smiths do their furnaces, with which the heart controls its respiration.[36]

It was as "a piece of craftsmanship deserving description above all others," that the author contemplated the usefulness of the heart's structure, its instrumentality. The evidence linking early anatomical inquiry with the belief in a preconceived plan is abundant and explicit.

And this makes sense. We don't try to interpret splashes of paint splattered on the floor by a cat. We simply rush to clean up "the mess." On the other hand, if we learn that the splashes were painted by a renowned artist, our view of them is suddenly transformed. Then they command reverent study, thoughtful regard. The presumption of divine design was absolutely critical to the enterprise of anatomy in just this way. It promised that a cadaver held more than frightening, repugnant gore — that its contents displayed visible meaning.

Greek intuitions of design in the world went back at least to the fourth century B.C.E.[37] Socrates attributes to Anaxagoras the theory that "mind produces order and is the cause of everything," and he takes this to mean that mind "arranges each individual thing in the way that is best for it."[38] In Xenophon's *Memorabilia*, Socrates himself counters Aristodemus' skepticism about the gods by appealing to the forethought manifest in the makeup of living creatures.[39] However, it was Plato's *Timaeus* that advanced the decisive analogy for the development of teleology — that relating the fashioning of the world to the work of the craftsman.

Here was a model that, on the one hand, made purpose central to creative expression and, on the other hand, explained that purpose in terms of a special mental seeing. Craftsmen "do not choose and apply their material to their work at random," Socrates contends, but work always "with the view that each of their productions should have a certain form (*eidos*)."[40] In making a table or couch, the craftsman "fixes his eyes on the idea, or form."[41] Creation is thus guided by an image; it is the act of translating imagined forms into matter. According to the myth of the *Timaeus*, this was also how the original demiurge worked. When he fashioned the world he kept a steady eye on "the pattern of the unchangeable."[42] It was this pattern, the forms envisioned by the creator, that defined the purpose of created things, their end. And it was these forms that the anatomist would eventually have to see.

125

Forms are hard to see, however. Plato himself never dissected, and moreover, he pointedly rejected what we normally call sight. True knowledge, he taught, has to be of what *is*, of unchanging Being; but the material world that our eyes apprehend is a world of perpetual flux, a realm of shadows, of simulacra, ceaselessly, at each moment, becoming something other. Rather than guiding us to eternal truths, our eyes delude and confuse. Hence Socrates's fear that he might blind his "soul altogether by observing objects with my eyes and trying to comprehend them with each of my other senses."[43] For when the soul uses the body "for any inquiry, whether through sight or hearing or any other sense — because using the body implies using the senses — it is drawn away by the body into the realm of the variable and loses its way and becomes confused and dizzy, as though it were befuddled."

Only "in that realm of the absolute, constant and invariable" — the realm of disembodied forms — is true wisdom possible.[44] In the allegory of the cave, the luminous vision of the Good is an experience not of the fleshly eye but of the immaterial soul, a metaphorical kind of seeing. Plato was the first, Friedlander tells us, to speak of "the eye of the soul" (*to tēs psychēs omma*) — the mind's eye.[45]

Aristotle's reinterpretation of forms, as something that the eye could directly see, helped bridge the transcendental speculations of the *Timaeus* with the actual inspection of animals.[46] Rather than a demiurge who forged all things of the cosmos, Aristotle touted Nature, an immanent force particularly shaping biological entities;[47] and whereas for Plato visible creation offered but dim glimmerings of the Ideal, Aristotle saw perfection in the creatures before our eyes. As intimated by his paradigm example of the bronze sphere (where the bronze is the matter and the sphere the form), "form" now frequently meant "visible shape."[48] *Eidos* was often interchangeable with *morphē*.[49] Form became inseparable from matter.

126

And yet, at the same time, form remained separate from matter. The metaphysical complexities of this ambiguous relation have been thoroughly explored by historians of philosophy. I should like to point out, however, that the tension between form and matter was also crucial for the history of dissection: it defined exactly the character of the anatomical gaze.

Aristotle concedes in an oft-cited passage of his *Parts of Animals* that "it is not possible without considerable disgust to look upon the blood, flesh, bones, blood vessels and similar parts of which the human body is constructed." [50] But he stresses that these aren't, in and of themselves, what anatomy is about. The anatomist yearns not for a look at the immediately sensible stuff of the body, which is repulsive, but rather for the contemplation (*theoria*) of Nature's purposive design.

As long as one trains one's eyes somehow to see beyond the matter of which animals are composed and to apprehend the whole configuration (*he holē morphē*) — the form as it reflects Nature's ends — then this gruesome enterprise of dissection can even be called beautiful. And it recommends itself to the philosopher by its convenience. For the divine realm of unchanging Being, which we all "long to learn about," eludes our senses. Plants and animals, on the other hand, because we live among them, can be studied more readily. This is the task of the scientist: to scrutinize these not in their perishable materiality but in their formal design, as refracted images of the divine. [51]

A sublime but subtle task. Dissection is never a straightforward uncovering of truths plain for all to see. It entails a special manner of seeing and requires an educated eye. The dissector must *learn* to discern order, through repeated practice, guided by teachers and texts. Without training and long experience, Galen insists, one sees nothing at all. [52] That is, one sees just a cadaver. And this doesn't count as anatomy — merely to pry open a corpse and stare blankly at bone and blood, fat, flesh, tangled tendons.

The anatomist aspires to see beyond the immediate, unpleasant material stuff of the body and behold the end (*telos*) for which each part is fashioned. "Rid your mind of the differences in material, and look at the pure art itself," exhorts Galen. Admire the form. Where the uninitiated see only opaque, meaningless matter, the true scientist (*technitēs*) marvels at how Nature, the great craftsman "does nothing in vain."[53]

This is why the history of anatomy cannot be summarized by bald tales of curiosity combating taboo. If at times religious restrictions braked or blocked the dissection of cadavers, the very impetus to anatomize represented, itself, a sort of spiritual desire.[54] Anatomy properly began when one learned to see through inchoate flesh and envision in *theoria* — "the eye of science," as A.L. Peck felicitously termed it — the purposive design. Seeing anatomically meant overcoming the blindness caused by the immediately visible. One had to see, and yet not see; see the form, but not the matter. See what, ultimately, can't be seen.[55]

Bodies mirrored souls and by this mirroring reflected the divine intelligence that shaped them. "I have frequently dissected such creeping animals as cats and mice, and crawling things, as the snake, and many kinds of birds and fishes," remarks Galen, "This I did to convince myself that there was a single mind that fashioned them, and that the body is suited in all ways to the character of the animal ... [E]ach animal has a bodily structure akin to the character and powers of the soul."[56] Each part of each creature manifested through its structure the use, that is, the function, for which it was conceived.

The model of the foresightful craftsman thus represented a certain theory of expression. Doctors gazed on the dissected body in a manner not unlike the way in which they listened to descriptions of the pulse. They scrutinized fleshly forms as sensible manifestations of insensible intent, much as they sought the motivating ideas behind words.

Chinese doctors, we know, listened to words rather differently, and in the next chapter we shall look at their vision of the expressive body. But we first must delve deeper into the topic at hand. The preceding inquiry into anatomical seeing represents just a start; our goal, remember, is to elucidate why in the West muscles came to appear so vivid, so intensely clear.

The Origins of the Muscular Body

The enigma of the muscular body actually encompasses two puzzles. One has to do with the origins of the interest in muscles; the other concerns the enchantment of what, to us, look like muscular bodies. Solving the first problem cannot fully resolve the second, because attraction to the "muscular" physique predated the widespread recognition of muscles.

To our eyes, the figures in the Parthenon metopes may look no less muscle-bound than Pollaiuolo's naked men. But this perception is anachronistic: almost certainly, the Greek artists who sculpted the former wouldn't have called their heroes muscular. The term "muscle" (*mys*) appears not at all in Homer, nor can it be found in Herodotus or Thucydides, or any of the dramatists. Plato, who was born after the completion of the Parthenon metopes, speaks extensively in the *Timaeus* of the flesh and sinews; but he, too, makes no mention of muscles. A sense of the body's muscularity emerged only gradually.

Hippocratic writers do refer to muscles, but remarkably sparingly. Even in those treatises where we might expect the closest scrutiny of musculature, such as the *Surgery* and *Fractures*, the preferred terms are *neuroi* and *sarks*, tendons/sinews and flesh. In language quite similar to what we find in China, the author of *Fractures* thus speaks of "bones, tendons, and *flesh*," rather than

129

"bones, tendons, and muscles"; and he cautions those treating the arm that the "fleshy growth" (*sarkos epiphysis*) over the radius is thick, while the ulna is almost fleshless.[57]

Muscles play no particular role in the Hippocratic conception of body. They are simply a kind of flesh. To the extent that muscles are distinguished from flesh — and the distinction is mentioned only rarely, and casually — the difference turns merely on degrees of firmness. The treatise *On the heart*, for instance, gives what at first blush reads like a modern definition, that is, the heart is a very strong muscle.[58] But it turns out that what makes it a muscle is only the closely pressed nature of its flesh (*pilēmati sarkos*; the verb *piloō* referred to the squeezing together of wool to make felt). This special density of construction equips the heart better to contain the innate heat.[59] Muscularity here had nothing to do with the post-Harveyian conception of the heart as a vigorous pump. *On Nutriment* identifies muscles in a similar way: except for tendons and bones, which are the hardest components, muscles are those body parts that are firmer and more resistant to dissolution than the rest.[60]

Sometime between Hippocrates and Galen, however, the traditional language of flesh and sinews became inadequate. It became common, and indeed indispensable, to speak of muscles. Whereas the plural *myes*, or muscles, appears just 14 times in the entire Hippocratic corpus, it figures over 460 times in Galen; and whereas in Hippocrates references to flesh outnumber references to muscles by roughly nine to one, in Galen they are about equal. In fact the contrast is even starker than such numbers suggest. Galen devoted entire books to the detailed, intensive study of these structures that Hippocratic physicians spoke of only rarely and in passing. And Galen wasn't alone, nor even the first. Galen himself tells us that serious study of muscles began with Marinus (first century c.e.), who discussed the subject at length in his treatise on anatomy. His disciples Pelops and Aelianus also wrote books on muscles, as did Lycus, son of Pelops, and one of Galen's teachers.[61]

There is a history to muscle-consciousness, then, a history framed, to repeat, by two problems. One concerns the nature of "muscular" bodies prior to the rise of muscle-consciousness. Greek artists represented figures with bulging ripples well before these ripples would have been identified as muscles, and they represented ripples even where, anatomically, no muscles exist. Yet if not as muscles, how did sculptors conceive these bulges they emphasized so? If not as indications of muscularity, what did Greek painters intend by the sharp demarcations lining the limbs and torsos of their men (figure 20)?

The second problem concerns the emergence of muscle-consciousness. Why did it eventually become necessary to speak of muscles in order to speak of the body? What prompted the keen interest in structures that previously laymen had not noticed at all, and that even physicians had scarcely recognized?

The issues are continuity and change. We must query muscularity as a concern that at once bridges and separates Galen's dissections and the metopes of the Parthenon. Although the sinuous ripples that early artists evoked for the eye, and the muscles about which later physicians composed treatises are surely related, just as surely they aren't identical. What did these ripples originally signify? And what change in consciousness transformed them into muscles?

With respect to the latter query, I've alluded already to one possible answer. I mean the rise of anatomy. We could guess that Hellenistic physicians spoke specifically of muscles rather than generically of flesh because, unlike their Hippocratic predecessors, they had probed below the surface. They had traced, and pulled apart, and observed distinct, individual muscles. The conti-

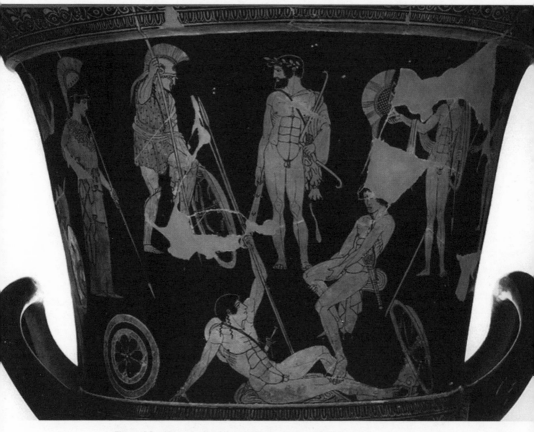

Figure 20. *Krater* by the Niobid painter, Louvre, Paris.

nuity and break between the classical and Hellenistic body thus might correspond simply to differing degrees of perspicuity. Early artists, we might suppose, saw the same structures that later anatomists saw, but vaguely and indistinctly — whence the general term "flesh" — while the latter grasped the shape and placement of each muscle with the clarity that comes only from dissecting the corpse.

This hypothesis would explain why a discourse of muscles began to thrive only after Hippocrates: systematic dissection, too, was a post-Hippocratic innovation. Galen's remark that muscles were an organ that "eluded discovery by observation and remained unknown" to Aristotle — "since he didn't take the pains to search for it by dissection" — would seem to strengthen the hypothesis.[62]

Yet as we noted above, and as Galen certainly knew, Aristotle was no stranger to dissection per se. Galen thus wasn't blaming Aristotle's ignorance of muscles on a general ignorance of anatomy. Muscles "remained unknown to" Aristotle in spite of the extensive dissections that he performed. Far from implying, in other words, that the discovery of muscles follows directly from the practice of anatomy, Galen's comment asserts that something more is necessary, that one has to take pains and search for muscles in order to observe them.

In sum, while the rise of anatomy undoubtedly contributed to nurturing muscle-consciousness, we would be wrong to regard the latter as an incidental by-product of the former. Rather than subsume the history of the muscular body under the history of dissection, I shall try to show, on the contrary, how a study of the muscular body alters our perspective on the anatomical imagination — how it beckons us to broaden our view of anatomical form, and invites us to see afresh, too, the bonds binding body and self.

The Aesthetics of Articulation

The fact that bulging ripples appear even in places where no muscles exist suggests that early artists aimed not so much to show specific structures as to give their figures a certain look. This point is crucial to interpreting "muscular" bodies prior to the discourse of muscles: the accent on rippling contours mirrored not least a sense of the beautiful.

What were the aesthetics of this physique? Wherein lay their appeal? How would Greek artists have described the look they so admired? I've explained that they wouldn't have called it "muscular." Yet they must have had other words to summon in speech the physique they displayed so magnificently for the eyes.

According to the *Physiognomics*, a pseudo-Aristotelian treatise on reading character from physique, strong character manifests itself in feet that are large, well-made, well-jointed and sinewy (*neurōdes*). A forceful character is also revealed in well-jointed and sinewy legs. Sinewy, clearly articulated ankles announce brave souls.[63] Here is an association we readily recognize — that between sinews and strength. We, too, perceive power in sinewy bodies.

Was it sinewiness of physiques like that of the discus thrower, then, that so fascinated the Greeks' gaze? Certainly, it must have been part of what people saw: references to the sinewy limbs of heroes are not uncommon. Notice though that the above readings of the body hearken as well, and repeatedly, to a less familiar, rather startling detail. It wasn't just in visible sinews that the *Physiognomics* discerned virtue: the feet, ankles, and legs of the strong and brave, we learn, are also well-jointed. Poorly-articulated (*anarthroi*) feet and ankles betray weakness and cowardice.

Despite its strangeness to us now, jointedness actually figures as a recurring theme in ancient appreciations of people. Nonmedical and medical writings alike draw attention to the presence or lack of articulation. In Sophocles' *Women of Trachis*, Hercules is borne on a litter, wracked in pain, exhausted and *anarthros* — literally, "without joints."[64] Euripides applies the same term to Orestes, as he lies prostrate, devastated by the experience of murdering his own mother.[65] To be *anarthros* was to be thoroughly debilitated, wasted. Orestes is barely alive, only faintly breathing; Heracles will soon die. These are men slumped in limp shapelessness. Sickness has melted their joints. Theirs are the precise opposite of those bodies adorning the Parthenon, the antithesis of the sharply articulated limbs and torsos of heroes in their prime, stretched taut in struggle, rippling with power.

Inarticulateness also marks the immature. Viviparous animals, Aristotle observes, produce offspring that from the start look similar to themselves, whereas other animals only produce something yet unarticulated (*adiarthrōtōn*), like eggs or larvae.[66] As for humans, the Hippocratic treatise *On the Seed* reports that a male fetus aborted before thirty days is still inarticulate (*anarthron*), whereas those aborted after thirty days have begun to articulate (*diēthrōmenai*).[67] The teleology of growth and development by which living things achieved their final form was a process of articulation.

Arthroi thus were not joints in the modern anatomical sense — at least, not just joints — but the divisions and differentiations that gave the body distinct form. Sometimes an articulation might well coincide with a joint: Oedipus is pierced through the "joints of his feet" (*arthroi podoin*), that is, through the ankles.[68] But Sophocles could also speak of the eyes that Oedipus gouges as the "joint of the globes" (*arthron tōn kyklōn*).[69] Mnesitheus, a physician of the third century B.C.E., refers to the internal organs as the "inner articulations" (*ta entos arthroi*).[70] Suggestively, the plural *arthroi*, by itself, regularly designated not joints, but the male and female genitals.[71]

Arthroi were also important in language: they were the words that partitioned the stream of discourse, what grammarians call articles.[72] Speech (*dialektos*) itself, the activity that made human beings truly human, was nothing other than "the articulation of voice by means of the tongue."[73] But the capacity to articulate the voice hinged, in turn, on possessing the right anatomical articulations — the organs of speech. This is the reason that Aristotle gives for why humans alone can speak. Insects and fish may produce sounds, but lacking a pharynx they have no voice. A dolphin has lungs and a windpipe and so has a voice, but "as its tongue cannot move freely, and as it has no lips, it cannot articulate the voice" (*ou . . . arthron to tēs phōnēs poein*);[74] it still can't speak.

Barbarians represented an interesting case. For though they had the necessary organs, some barbarian peoples seemed scarcely more articulate than animals. Strabo's etymology of *barbaros*, "barbaric," as onomatopoeic for the barking of dogs — or so foreign speech sounded to Greek ears — springs to mind.[75] Diodorus of Sicily, for his part, describes a primitive tribe known as the Fish Eaters, who gorge themselves on fish, then merrily entertain each other with "inarticulate songs."[76] "But the most surprising thing of all," according to Diodorus, "is that in lack of sensibility they surpass all men, and to such a degree that what is recounted of them is scarcely credible."[77]

> Indeed, when a man drew his sword and brandished it at them they did not turn to flight, nor, if they were subjected to insult or even to blows, would they show irritation, and the majority were not moved to anger in sympathy with the victims of such treatment; on the contrary, when at times children or women were butchered before their eyes they remained insensible in their attitudes, displaying no sign of anger or, on the other hand, of pity. In short, they remained unmoved in the face of the most appalling horrors, looking stead-

fastly at what was taking place and nodding their heads at each incident. Consequently, they say, they speak no language, but by movements of the hands ... they point out everything they need.[78]

The Fish Eaters have no language, and only gesticulate. Note that Diodorus introduces this observation with the word "consequently" (*dio*), implying that the ability to speak requires the ability to feel — to distinguish what is dangerous, or injust, or cruel. Aristotle held that sensitivity, too, was a function of anatomical articulation. "The articulations of the heart," he observes in *Parts of Animals*, "are more distinct in animals whose sensation is keen, and less distinct in the duller ones, such as swine."[79]

The image of the inarticulate savage who can only grunt, or bark, or gesture wildly is familiar. But the Greek conception of barbarian inarticulacy also had a more concrete aspect: sometimes their very bodies lacked clear joints and divisions. The Hippocratic treatise *Airs, Waters, Places*, for instance, reports that the nomadic Scythians roam lands where

> the changes of the seasons are neither great nor violent, the seasons being uniform and altering but little. Wherefore the men are also like one another in physique, since summer and winter they always use similar food and the same clothing, breathing a moist, thick atmosphere, drinking water from ice and snow, and abstaining from fatigue. For neither bodily or mental endurance is possible where the changes are not violent. Because of these causes their physiques are gross, fleshy, inarticulate (*anarthra*), moist and flabby....[80]

The Scythians, in short, lack differentiation — both among themselves and within each body. Because they experience little seasonal change they all resemble each other and lack individuality. Because they breathe moist mist and drink icy water, their bodies are moist and flabby and lack definition. Furthermore, in them, as in the exhausted Orestes and the dying Hercules, inarticulateness signals weakness. The Scythians are a people wanting in bodily and mental endurance.

It is to compensate for their natural debility, the Hippocratic author explains, that the Scythians cauterize themselves on the arms, wrists, breast, hips, and loins: "For owing to their moistness and flabbiness they have not the strength either to draw a bow or to throw a javelin from the shoulder. But when they have been cauterized, the excess of moisture dries up from their joints, and their bodies become more braced (*entonōtera*), more nourished and better articulated."[81] Cautery dries the joints, articulates the body, makes it firm. Cautery is a form of bodybuilding. But bodybuilding for what end? The Greek reporter immediately thinks: to enable the throwing of the javelin and the drawing of the bow.

We might suppose that the pleasure with which the Greeks lingered on the articulated physique was related to their admiration of athletes and warriors; related, too, to their keen interest in *agon*, in struggle, in those moments of tense effort when sinewy demarcations surface most sharply. But to judge these connections justly we must bear two points in mind.

One is the artificiality of the highly articulated body: it is and was the product of extreme and sustained exertions. The physiques of bodybuilders today are often compared with, and of course the bodybuilders themselves strive consciously to emulate, the sharply defined, "muscular" physiques seen in Greek sculptures. But to achieve such physiques even the most naturally gifted of contemporary bodybuilders must pursue an extraordinary regimen of punishing exercise, fueled by the consumption of prodigious amounts of food.[82] There is no reason to suppose that Greek athletes had it any easier, that they were naturally blessed with their admired physiques. No ordinary life — even a physically vigorous one of soldiering or tilling the fields — could have created the bulk and definition of a body like that of Hercules (figure 21).

Greek doctors and philosophers voiced qualms about both the process and the consequences of this extreme discipline. Hippocratic treatises warned that athletes endangered their health by, paradoxically, being in "too good a condition." For such a condition couldn't persist for long, and since it couldn't change for the better, it would change for the worse.[83] Besides objecting on philosophical grounds to their preoccupation with the body (and consequent neglect of the soul), Plato also criticized athletic disciplines as "precarious for health." For "if they depart ever so little from their prescribed regimen," he observed, "these athletes are liable to great and violent diseases."[84] And of course there were moral perils as well: devotees of gymnastics might well be high-spirited and brave, but if their training was not counterbalanced by education in music, these men became brutally hard and harsh.[85]

Yet if the athletic physique was sculpted only through the most extraordinary effort — and if, moreover, the result of this effort was a body that was exceptionally vulnerable to sickness and a character prone to brutality — wherein lay its appeal? I've already mentioned the rich fabric of ideals woven around articulation. But we musn't forget another, compelling factor: the stress on strength and struggle and the hard, spare physique reflected an acute consciousness of their opposites.

If Plato decried the harshness that single-minded devotion to physical training could produce, he worried no less about the softening influences of music. For a man who abandons himself exclusively to music, "melts and liquefies till he completely dissolves away his spirit, cuts out as it were the very sinews of his soul and makes of himself a 'feeble warrior.'"[86] Though Plato called for a balance of "relaxation and tension,"[87] Greek writers

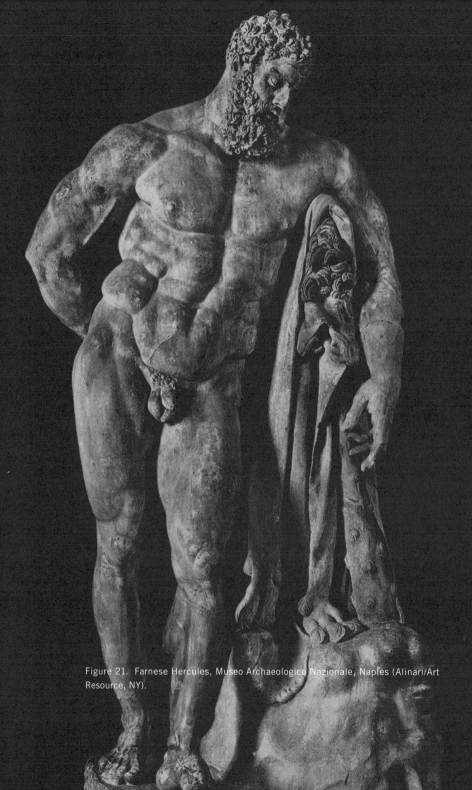

Figure 21. Farnese Hercules, Museo Archaeologico Nazionale, Naples (Alinari/Art Resource, NY).

often evinced special anxieties about softness, a distinct preference for the hard.

When it was proposed to King Cyrus that the Persians abandon their barren homeland and move to the fertile plains they had conquered, the Persian king replied,

> that they might act upon it if they pleased, but added the warning that, if they did so, they must prepare themselves to rule no longer, but to be ruled by others. "Soft countries," he said, "breed soft men. It is not the property of any one soil to produce fine fruits and good soldiers too." The Persians had to admit that this was true and that Cyrus was wiser than they; so they left him, and chose rather to live in a rugged land and rule than to cultivate rich plains and be subject to others.[88]

So concludes the *Histories* of Herodotus. Herodotus put the speech in the mouth of King Cyrus, but the sentiments were at least as Greek as they were Persian. The difference between firm bodies and soft bodies was the divide between rulers and slaves.

Airs, Waters, Places echoed the contrast. "Where the land is rich, soft, and well-watered," we learn, "there the inhabitants are fleshy, ill-articulated (*anarthroi*), moist, lazy, and generally cowardly in nature." But where "the land is bare, waterless, rough, oppressed by winter's storms and burnt by the sun, there you will see men who are hard, lean, well-articulated (*diērthrōmenous*), well-braced, and hairy; such natures will be found energetic, vigilant, stubborn, and independent in character and temper, wild rather than tame, of more than average sharpness and intelligence in the arts, and in war of more than average courage."[89]

Europe encompassed both hard and soft environments, includes both hard and soft peoples. But comparatively speaking, the Hippocratic author asserted, the opposition of the articulated

141

and the inarticulate, of the brave and pusillanimous, corresponded to the divide between Europe and Asia.

Because seasonal change is more violent in Europe than in Asia, the European physique varies more than the Asian. The Asian physique and character largely replicates the Scythian. Shaped like the Scythians by a climate with little seasonal variation, Asians resemble each other, their bodies lack articulation and their spirits want endurance. Europeans, by contrast, "are more courageous than Asiatics. For uniformity engenders slackness, while variation fosters endurance in both body and soul. Rest and slackness are food for cowardice, endurance and exertion for bravery. Wherefore the Europeans are more warlike...."[90] The taut, lean bodies of Europe were the bodies of hardy conquerors. The individualized, articulated physique embodied European identity.

Visible joints, in short, separated one part of the body from another, distinguished individuals from each other, divided Europeans from Asians. To this list we must add one more: visible joints demarcated male from female. According to Hippocratic embryology, if the male fetus takes thirty days to begin articulating, the female fetus, being more moist, takes forty-two.[91] More generally, males are fiery and dry, females are moist and cold. But the solid parts of body, like the sinews and bones, are formed by fire drying out the original moisture.[92] In the hermeneutics of the *Physiognomics*, the fleshy, poorly jointed feet, ankles, and legs that signal weak and cowardly characters, are the feet and ankles and legs typical of women. Sinewy, well-jointed limbs are characteristic of men.[93]

But what about Scythian men? They are male, but also flabby barbarians. It is the latter that proves decisive. The great majority of Scythian men, *Airs, Waters, Places* reports, "become impotent, do women's work, and live like women, and talk like women."[94] "Because of the moistness of their constitution, and the softness

and chill of their abdomen, they have no great desire for intercourse."[95] In their lack of passion, as in the formlessness of their
bodies, they are like castrated eunuchs who, in the words of the
pseudo-Aristotelian *Problems*, change into the likeness of the female, developing a female voice, and shapelessness (*amorphian*)
and inarticulation (*anarthrian*).[96]

Central, then, to the ethics and aesthetics of the "muscular"
physique before the rise of muscle-consciousness was the virtue
of articulation. Before they became fascinated with special structures named muscles, the Greeks celebrated bodies that had a
particular look — a special clarity of form, a distinct "jointedness,"
which they identified with the vital as opposed to the dying, the
mature as opposed to the yet unformed, individuals as opposed to
people who all resemble each other, the strong and brave as opposed to the weak and cowardly, Europeans as opposed to Asians,
the male as opposed to the female.

Muscularity and Agency

So how did this well-articulated body become the muscular body?
We come to our second question, that of the origins of muscle-
consciousness.

I said before that the rise of anatomy likely assisted this development, and I pointed out how we owe the earliest extended
discussions of muscles to renowned dissectors of the first and
second centuries c.e. — Marinus, Aelianus, Pelops, Lycus, and
above all Galen. But I also cautioned against exaggerating the role
of anatomical observation. For if we conceive muscles simply as
structures that dissectors saw, that is, as mere objects of visual
knowledge, we risk overlooking the one definitive characteristic
of the new discourse on muscularity: whereas physicians previously spoke of flesh chiefly in describing how the body *looked*,
they now invoked muscles to understand how the body *worked*.

Muscles, in other words, were not just flesh perceived with enhanced perspicuity; they were unique organs invested with a unique
function.

Galen observes that some processes in the body go on without
our attending to them, and we can't directly influence them even
if we wish. Such is the case with digestion and pulsation. But
there are also activities, like walking and talking, that hinge on
our desires and intentions. We can choose to walk faster, or slow
down, stand still. We can alter the cadence of our speech. We can
do all these things, Galen explains, because we have these organs
called muscles. This is what muscles are: "the organs of voluntary
motion."[97] Muscles allow us to choose what we do, and when, and
how; and this choice marks the divide between voluntary actions
and involuntary processes. Muscles, in short, identify us as genuine agents.

 I come to my chief contention about the origins of muscle-
consciousness: the rise of the preoccupation with muscles, I suggest, is inextricably intertwined with the emergence of a particular
conception of personhood. Specifically, in tracing the crystallization of the concept of muscle, we are also, and not coincidentally, tracing the crystallization of the sense of an autonomous will.
Interest in the muscularity of the body was inseparable from a preoccupation with the agency of the self.

This is why Galen's treatise, *On the Movement of Muscles*, goes
far beyond an exposition of muscular function, and struggles with
the conundrums of action and self-awareness. How can we explain, after all — if human beings are muscular creatures and muscles are the organs of voluntary motion — the man who sings in
drunken stupor or walks in his sleep?[98] These actions obviously
involve the work of many muscles. Yet those performing them
seem to have no consciousness of performing them.

Nor are the puzzles confined to quirks like sleepwalking. They appear even in the most quotidian activities. Thus, the philosopher who walks from Piraeus to Athens lost in thought may have no recollection of the road, or of attending to his arms and feet. And people absorbed in conversation or debate often display mannerisms of which they themselves are unaware. The way in which the soul acts in and through the body, Galen admits, isn't always transparent.[99] But he adamantly insists that it acts all the same.

Just consider: if all the various muscles were to give way to their natural tendency to contract — a tendency easily demonstrated by cutting the tendon at one end of a muscle — they would counteract each other, and the body would lock into tetanoid immobility. That such immobility is exceptional, the very fact of our habitual mobility, proves that another force is also at work, some psychic power (*psychikē dynamis*). Another example: the arm of someone whose extensor muscles are severed flexes automatically due to the contraction of the flexor muscles. But the person can actually flex even further, that is, contract the flexors beyond their state of natural contraction, simply by deciding to do so. Complete flexion requires the action of the soul.[100]

The life of a person cannot be told, therefore, merely in terms of natural processes like digestion and the pulsing of the arteries. Beyond processes that happen of themselves, there are also the actions willed by the soul and carried out by these instruments called muscles. Because our attention is spotty, however, this psychic intervention isn't always apparent; we are acutely aware of doing certain things, others we may have no memory of having done at all. Yet even the mere acts of sitting or standing, Galen argues, even apparent nonactivity, are genuine acts. They engage the so-called tonic action (*tonikē kinēsis*) of muscles. Our ability to sustain a given posture is only possible because of the active tensing of a host of muscles. Remove the living soul and the statuesque poised person in figure 2 melts into limp inarticulate flesh.

145

Jean-Pierre Vernant observes that in Homer the body doesn't stand isolated and independent, shut up in itself, but "is fundamentally permeable to the forces that animate it, accessible to the intrusion of the vital powers that make it act. When a man feels joy, irritation or pity, when he suffers, is bold or feels any emotion he is inhabited by drives... which, *breathed into him by a god*, run through and across him like a visitor coming from the outside" (italics added).[101]

Considered together with the preceding remarks on muscles and volition, Vernant's analysis of archaic conceptions of embodiment suggest one possible reason why, even in Hippocrates' time, figural representations of what we see as muscularity weren't accompanied by a discourse of muscles. The bulging swells that knot the limbs and torsos of mythical beasts and heroes may signal courage, or strength, or passion; but in contemplating these signs we must keep in mind the old tradition that envisioned strength and passion and all the virtues of heroes not as personal qualities rooted in an inner self, but as marks of divine favor, manifesting the influx of godly powers.[102]

By the fifth century B.C.E, to be sure, we are starting to enter a different world. By the end of the century, Socrates will be speaking of human beings as creatures centered around an immortal core called the soul. But it would still take time for the Socratic soul, a prisoner in flesh, fully to evolve into Galen's autonomous agent — into a self possessing muscular will.

Seventeenth-century physiologists would cite Galen as their source for the definition of muscles as the instruments of the will. But Galen didn't invent the formula: we encounter it before him in Rufus of Ephesus.[103] Moreover, we've noted that Galen himself cites the anatomist Marinus as the founder of myology, and we know that Marinus' treatise on anatomy included a discussion of voluntary movements.

146

We can go back earlier still. Although Aristotle doesn't mention muscles in analyzing the movements of animals, he does distinguish between those movements that are *hekousious*, motivated by choice or desire, like the making of a house or cloak, and those that are *akousious*, which occur even if we don't consciously choose them, like the movements of the heart and penis, sleep and waking, respiration.[104] His distinction obviously resembles Galen's later opposition of voluntary and involuntary movements, and may underlie Galen's cryptic suggestion that, though Aristotle never observed nor knew muscles, he nonetheless knew them *in theory*.[105] Still, there are revealing differences.

Consider again the theme of articulation. Language, the articulation of voice, requires a certain anatomy; but beyond that, self-mastery too is essential. Which is why very young infants can't speak. For, Aristotle explains, "just as they have not proper control over their limbs generally, so [infants] cannot at first control their tongue, which is imperfect and attains complete freedom of motion later on; until then, they mumble and lisp for the most part."[106] Articulation is thus a matter of function as well as of structure, a relationship between the person and the body. Infants can only mumble and lisp, and cannot speak, because they cannot yet control their tongue, move it as they wish.

For Aristotle, however, this relationship between the person and the body constitutes just part of a longer chain of causation. Movement can never be fully explained by the disposition and desires of the person here and now. The possibility of the simplest actions — the opening and closing of our eyes, for example — is rooted in a past prior to consciousness, prior even to birth, when Nature first shaped the embryo:

> Since Nature does nothing in vain, the separation of the eyelids and
> the ability to move them must coincide in time. Thus the comple-

tion of the formation of the eyes comes late, because of the large amount of concoction required by the brain, and it comes last, after all the other parts, because the movement must be very strong and powerful in order to move parts which are so far away from the first principle, and so much subjected to cold. That such is the nature of the eyelids is shown by the fact that even if a very little heaviness affects the head through sleep or intoxication or anything of that sort, we are unable to raise the eyelids though their weight is very slight.[107]

Why are we unable, sometimes, when we are sleepy or drunk, to resist even the feathery fall of our eyelids? Aristotle sought an essential part of the answer in the original process by which the innate pneuma (*symphyton pneuma*), the fiery divine breath of Nature, spread out from the heart (the first principle), articulating the moist embryo, and finally separating the eyelids.

His understanding of just how the aetherial heavens relate to animal motions isn't entirely clear, but there is no doubt that he felt this relationship to be vital.[108] And in this conviction we glimpse the distance that still separates his account of animation from the muscular volition that so fascinated Galen. Georges Canguilhem contrasts them this way:

> For Aristotle, all movement depends on a primal unmoved mover. All movement in nature hangs, by respiration and by imitation, upon a supernatural act. In the most perfect terrestrial animal, the human being, there is a soul which enters the embryo from the outside, and which derives from the divine ether, the soul of the stars....

> For Galen, motion is truly the expression of an internal spontaneity. ... Thus, in Galen's conception, the motion of the living being is the effect of a force immanent in the organism. The animal ... moves

itself in its environment...The animal, in its muscular movements, propels itself from its own center.[109]

Canguilhem's remarks gesture toward yet another way to construe the origins of muscle-consciousness — in terms of a shift from a teleology of cosmic motion to the spontaneous movements of autonomous agents.

In discussing the history of the touch, I stressed how the manner in which we perceive something owes much to what we imagine the thing to be. But, in the case of the body, that imagined object is none other than ourselves, and the problem of modes of seeing merges into the issue of personal identity. The history of the Greek muscular body involved, early on, the history of how Greek men defined themselves vis-à-vis various Others — animals, barbarians, women. But it subsequently became entwined as well with the evolution of another, less-studied aspect of self-definition, namely, the relationship of the self to change. The obsession with muscles reflected the birth of a new experience of embodied life and an altered perception of persons. Henceforth, the heart of all readings of the body would be framed by the dichotomy opposing processes that merely happen, naturally or by chance, and actions initiated by the soul.

The Hippocratic treatise *On the Heart*, recall, identified the heart as "a very strong muscle" — which of course coincides with the modern view. And so it may appear paradoxical that in the period after Hippocrates, precisely when anatomy and the discourse of muscularity truly blossomed, Greek doctors seemingly regressed and ceased to consider the heart as a muscle. The paradox is easily explained. In the treatise *On the Heart*, the notion of muscle is as yet vague; the heart is called a muscle simply because of its densely compressed flesh. For Galen, the crux of muscularity would be function. The heart isn't a muscle because it moves of its own accord, because it isn't an instrument of the will. We cannot start or stop it as we want.[110]

Reflect back now to chapter 1, and we see the birth of pulse diagnosis in a new light. Greek doctors like Alexander and Demosthenes, remember, defined the pulse as "the *involuntary* contraction of the heart and the arteries." Before them, Herophilus launched the whole enterprise of sphygmology by drawing attention to the pulse as something that "*exists naturally and attends us involuntarily* at all times." Underlying his isolation of the pulse as something radically different from tremors and spasms was the separation of the heart and the arteries from the "nervelike" (*to neurōdes*) parts of the body — specifically, the nerves, muscles, and tendons. For Herophilus, this anatomical partition corresponded to a basic duality in human life: whereas the movements of the nervelike parts were subject to intentional choice (*prohairesis*), the pulsations of the heart and arteries lay beyond conscious control.[111]

"I once allowed someone to hold a heart with a smith's tongs," Galen relates, "since it jumped out of his fingers because of the violent palpitation; but even then the animal suffered no impairment of sensation or voluntary movement. It uttered a loud scream, breathed without hindrance, and kept all its limbs in violent motion ... Once these facts have been established, another more important fact comes to light as a consequence, that the heart does not need the brain at all for the exercise of its proper movement, nor the brain the heart."[112]

Such separation of powers was the central thesis of Galen's treatise *On the Doctrines of Plato and Hippocrates*. Galen sought not so much to decide between the supremacy of the brain and the supremacy of the heart, but rather to demonstrate the existence of two distinct and independent (though, of course, interacting) functions: feeling, located in the heart, and willing and sensing, located in the brain. The problem with the cardiocentric theory was not just its single-minded emphasis on the heart, but its undifferentiated view of human psychology.

Herophilus' opposition of the nervelike parts to the heart and arteries didn't immediately carry the day. Many even in Galen's time still followed Aristotle and Chrysippus in locating not just emotions, but speech, judgment, and will in the heart. Thus, they marvel, says Galen, "when suddenly they hear that speech comes from the brain, and they marvel even more and call us posers of paradoxes when they hear that all voluntary movements are produced by muscles."[113] The persistence of such attitudes presumably underlies Galen's comment that "the limbs are moved by the muscles, *as they are called (hoi de onomazomenoi myes)*," as if the very notion of muscle had yet to be universally accepted and taken for granted.[114]

In a sense, then, the fixation on muscles and the birth of pulse diagnosis represented the obverse and reverse faces of a single development. We can comprehend neither except by pondering the emergence of a fundamental schism in Western self-understanding: the split between voluntary actions and natural processes. The pulse revealed nothing, as John Donne would later lament, about sin and redemption and the state of the eternal soul. Nor did it display the soul's decisions. But it expressed, on the other hand, the large realm of human existence on which nature *could* lay claim — all the changes, physiological and pathological, beyond the reach of volition, the impulses and yearnings, like prince Antiochus' forbidden passion, that move a person regardless of the will.

CHAPTER FOUR

The Expressiveness of Colors

> The main fact, then, about a flower is that it is the part of
> the plant's form developed at the moment of its intensest
> life; and this inner rapture is usually marked externally for
> us by the flush of one or more of the primary colors.
> — John Ruskin, *Queen of the Air*

Doctors in China missed much of the detail observed by Greek dissectors and incorporated invisible features that dissection could never justify. This especially is what makes the acupuncture man seem a mystery — the blind indifference to the claims of anatomy.

Yet indifference to anatomy didn't mean a slighting of the eyes. Not at all: ancient Chinese doctors evinced great faith in visual knowledge. Like their Greek counterparts, they scrutinized the body intently. Only they somehow saw it differently.

Declared the *Nanjing*: to gaze and know the illness is "divine" (*shen*), to know by listening or smelling is "sagely" (*sheng*), to question and know was "crafty" (*gong*), to touch and know only "skillful" (*qiao*).[1] Divine insight thus crowned the hierarchy of diagnostic means. The *Lingshu* ranked perceptual skills slightly differently, but it too gave priority to the "enlightened" (*ming*)

153

gaze.[2] The *Shanghanlun* was blunt: the physician who knew by gazing belonged to the top class (*shanggong*); the physician who questioned and knew was average (*zhonggong*); the physician who touched and knew was inferior (*xiagong*).[3] Mastery of medicine was defined first by an exceptional eye.

Consider the legend of Bian Que, the most celebrated name in the history of Chinese medicine. Originally, we are told, Bian Que had no connection to the healing arts. He was managing a boarding house when, one day, an aged boarder named Chang-sang Jun drew him aside. "I possess secret skills," the guest confided, "but I am old, and want to pass them on." Producing an elixir, Changsang Jun advised, "Drink this with fresh dew for thirty days, and you will know things." Bian Que did as he was told, and soon discovered that he could see through walls and inside bodies.[4]

Penetrating insight was thus key to his transformation into "the Hippocrates of China." Bian Que's name became synonymous with medical acumen partly because he could see, literally, what others could not. In his celebrated diagnosis of Duke Huan, Bian Que tracks the progress of the duke's malady not by questioning him, or smelling or touching him, but just by peering at him from a distance. (More on this diagnosis below.)

Scholars have sometimes spoken of the hegemony of the visual as a peculiarly Western trait.[5] And it is true that epistemological discourse in Europe long conflated seeing and knowing, sight and perception, observation and experience, *autopsia* and *empeiria*. Greek terms like *noos*, *idea*, and *eidos*, we noted before, cast the very act of thinking as a kind of envisioning.

But any bare contrast pitting visual against nonvisual traditions is too crude. Chinese philosophers, for their part, spoke of the obscurity (*xuan*) and the fine-grained subtlety (*wei*) of the Way, and of the brightness (*ming*) of intelligence, and of contemplating (*guan*) cosmic principles. And the evidence of the *Nanjing* and the Bian Que legend testifies to how in Chinese medicine, too, sight claimed privileged status.

Of course, this evidence also intimates a telling difference: visual knowledge in Chinese medicine was mostly a matter of *diagnostic* sight. It engaged a gaze trained on living persons rather than on lifeless corpses. This accordingly is the main focus of what follows — how Chinese doctors scrutinized the living.

But I want to start with how they inspected the dead. Though anatomy in China never gained dominance as a way of understanding the body, it certainly wasn't unknown.[6] In *Lingshu* treatise 12 the minister Qi Bo expostulates to the Yellow Emperor about what can be learned by "dissecting and inspecting"; and the *Hanshu* biography of Wang Mang records that in 16 C.E. a dissection was actually performed. Both passages are brief, and together they represent the only explicit references to medical anatomy in ancient China.[7] Still, they are enlightening.

Hints of an Alternative Anatomy

> Wangsun Qing, the confederate of Zhai Yi, was captured. Wang Mang sent his personal Palace Physician and artisans from the Directorate for Imperial Manufactories to work with skilled butchers to dissect Wangsun. They measured and weighed his five solid viscera, and used a bamboo strip to trace the courses of his mo to learn where they began and ended. [The Emperor] said [this knowledge] could be used to cure illness.[8]

Wangsun Qing was allied with Wang Mang's defeated rival, the rebel Zhai Yi; and from this circumstance, Mikami Yoshio hypothesized half a century ago that there was a punitive aspect to this dissection.[9] The possibility can't be ruled out. It wouldn't have been the first time that curiosity and cruelty worked in concert. When the vicious tyrant Zhou captured Bi Gan, he reportedly mused, "I've heard that the heart of a sage has seven orifices" and ordered the rebel cut open to check.[10] But Mikami's hypothesis suffers from the difficulty that the *Hanshu* account itself breathes not a word about vengeance, and that the procedures it recounts betray no malice. We are directed explicitly, instead, to another goal: acquiring insights useful in healing.

Was this the prime motive for the dissection, or just an incidental benefit recognized along the way? The passage doesn't say. In any event, it is an extraordinary expectation. Beginning students of gross anatomy know how frustratingly elusive even major structures can seem, even today, with the help of teachers, modern atlases, and dissecting manuals that guide one step by step. Yet the dissection of Wangsun Qing was ostensibly the first, and quite possibly the only dissection ever conducted in ancient China. We would have expected to find the dissectors less sure about how to proceed; but the *Hanshu* account betrays no uncertainty. On the contrary, it evinces a remarkable confidence about both the method of investigation and the usefulness of the resulting knowledge. The dissectors knew exactly what they wanted to know. Apparently without hesitating, they moved straight to measuring and weighing the viscera, and tracing the course of blood vessels.

Lingshu treatise 12 sheds some light on the logic of these procedures. The height of the heavens, the breadth of the earth, Qi Bo declares, these transcend what human beings can measure. By contrast, the human body is directly accessible and of modest proportions. One can measure along its surface; and after death one can dissect. By dissection one determines the consistency of the *zang* (solid viscera), the size of the *fu* (hollow viscera), their capacity for grain, the length of the vessels, the clarity or turbidity of the blood and its amount, which vessels have more blood and less qi, and which vessels the reverse. All these have their norm, their measure (*dashu*).[11]

We are reminded of Aristotle's apology for anatomy. In *Parts of Animals*, recall, this pioneer of Greek dissection urged us to study plants and animals because they are close at hand, whereas heavenly Being, which we all yearn to know, lies beyond the reach of our senses. Qi Bo, for his part, contrasts the unknowable immensity of the universe to the finite measurable body, and hints that we might yet glimpse the former in the latter. Just before this passage he had already related each of the major conduits of the body to one of the large rivers of China. It is in response to the Yellow Emperor's query about the practical application of such correspondences — about how they should guide the depth of needle insertion or the number of moxa cones to burn — that Qi Bo expounds the meaning and uses of dissection.

Like Aristotle, then, Qi Bo approached anatomy as a sort of cosmic inquiry. But he scrutinized details that the Aristotelian gaze, fixed on design, the form as it displayed Nature's ends, ignored. Qi Bo sought to take the measure of the body, to know its numbers.

The phrase *dashu*, "great number," hearkened to the heavenly regularities discovered by the astronomer, the secrets of the diviner. No blind chance matched the number of a person's limbs with the four seasons and the four directions, the five zang with the five planets, the twelve conduits streaming through the body with the twelve rivers bearing life to the land of the Central Kingdom. The dissection of Wangsun Qing took place in a culture where numbers confirmed the resonance between macrocosm and microcosm and summarized the lawful orderliness of the world.

Yet the anatomical dimensions actually cited in the *Neijing* and *Nanjing* don't reverberate with any obvious cosmic design. Nor do these texts attempt to interpret them in that way. If faith in numerical correspondences helped to rationalize Chinese dissection, it doesn't appear to have predetermined the findings. The numbers are too diverse and precise. They read like real records.[12]

The skull measures 26 *cun* around, the circumference of the chest is 45 *cun*, and around the waist is 42 *cun*. From the top of the head to the nape of the neck is 12 *cun*. From the hair down to the chin is 10 *cun*.[13] By measuring the girths, widths, and lengths of the bones and joints, we are told, one can also fix the length of the moving vessels. These are some of the easier measurements — those taken at the body surface.

Other calculations are more involved. The mouth, the *Lingshu* reckons, is 2.5 *cun* wide; from the teeth to the back of the throat is 3.5 *cun*; the capacity of the oral cavity is 5 *he*. The tongue weighs 10 *liang*; it is 5 *cun* long and 2.5 *cun* wide. The stomach weighs 2 *jin*, 2 *liang*; it is 2 *chi*, 6 *cun* long, and measures 1 *chi*, 5 *cun* in circumference; its capacity is 3 *dou*, 5 *sheng*. The bladder weighs 9 *liang*, 2 *zhu*; it is 9 *cun* wide, and its capacity is 9 *liang*, 9 *he*. The list goes on.[14]

These probably were not averages calculated from the inspection of many corpses. The absence of other references to anatomy in ancient China argues against that. Moreover, the several texts that list anatomical dimensions mostly repeat the same results, hinting that the cited numbers may well have all derived from the one dissection of Wangsun Qing.[15] At the same time, though, this one dissection was clearly a serious investigation. The nature of the measurements compels us to picture a systematic, time-consuming process, with the dissectors isolating and cutting out each organ, spreading it out, gauging it against scales, then tying up an opening, then filling the organ with grain or water, then emptying the grain and water, then weighing, measuring, calculating.

Why did they bother? What did they hope to learn? We've noted the belief in cosmic correspondences. The method manifest in the dissection, however, suggests another possible inspiration. I mean the ethos of the unified state.

The first Qin emperor pursued an ambitious program of standardization, specifying the metal contents of coins, the width of wheel axles, the breadth of roads; he decreed universal measures of length and weight, prescribed a simplified uniform script, and tried, most notoriously, to sear minds clean of heterodoxy by burning heterodox books. And though the last act was widely reviled, rulers of subsequent dynasties continued to stress set standards. When the Yellow Emperor says in *Lingshu* treatise 14, "I would like to hear about the dimensions of commoners. What are the girths and lengths of the bone and joints in someone seven and a half *chi* tall?"[16] we can hear the voice of a Staatswissenschaft intent on framing human diversity within numerical norms.

The dissection of Wangsun Qing was a rare, perhaps unique exception. Overall, anatomical inspection left only faint impressions on the ancient Chinese conception of the body. Nonetheless, the exception reinforces an important lesson of the previous chapter, namely, that there is more than one way to cut open the body and look, that what we habitually call anatomy is just *one kind* of anatomy.[17] When dissectors inspected the body in ancient China they didn't see the nerves and muscles that Greek anatomists found so arresting. They lingered instead on measurements that Galen and his predecessors entirely ignored.[18]

On the Notion of Somatic Structure

Yet what of the functional connections between the viscera measured with such care, the unity of the body as a whole? Greek anatomy aimed not least to show the structure of somatic government, to elucidate how centers like the brain and the heart ruled the periphery — the muscles, the pulsing arteries. If the investigations recorded in the *Hanshu* somehow don't seem like "real" anatomy, it is largely because they appear indifferent to the *uses* of the parts that they measure, unconcerned about how the body *works*.

Plainly, this isn't entirely true. Dissectors tried after all to trace the course of the *mo* with bamboo strips, to measure their lengths, to check the clarity or turbidity of the blood in each, to gauge which had more blood and less *qi*, and which the reverse — and all this, surely, because the ties defined by the *mo* had functional meaning. The *mo* that ran through the liver flowed into the eyes; hence the link between liver weakness and faltering sight. The *mo* that rose up from the foot and up through the gall bladder made its way up the side of the body, coiled around the ears and then entered them; this was why one treated the gall bladder for dizziness and ringing in the ears. Much like the nerves and blood vessels of Western anatomy, the *mo* linked the fates of distant parts.

Unlike the nerves and blood vessels, though, the *mo* formed a circle with no controlling source. Palpation of the *mo* gave insight into all the viscera equally, not just or even primarily the heart. Circulation began from and returned to simply a place, the *cunkou*, the inch-opening at the wrist;[19] it had no originating motor, no prime mover.

Here Chinese intuitions diverged fundamentally from the Greek. Even before the rise of anatomy, Greek reflections on the body highlighted the question, Where is its ruling principle (*archē*), its controller (*hegemonikon*)? And though opinions varied — Plato and Diogenes championed the supremacy of the brain, while others like Aristotle pushed the heart's hegemony — all took the problem for granted. The motions within a person had to spring from some ultimate source. There had to be a ruler.

The eventual concentration of intense anatomical interest in the brain and in the heart owed much to this preoccupation with origins. Greek dissectors assumed, as a matter of course, that this was what understanding the body's structure was largely about — elucidating the structure of control. Galen, in his anatomy, postulated a three-part division of power, as he traced the nerves to the brain, the arteries to the heart, the veins to the liver; but the problem of ultimate rule remained central to his thinking. The three sources were by no means equal: as the seat of reason, the brain reigned supreme.

No comparable hegemon governed the Chinese body. To be sure, when the *Neijing* drew parallels between the body and the body politic, it did speak of the heart as the ruling lord (*junzhu zhi guan*), and it even endowed the heart with intelligence (*shenming*). But the heart hardly monopolized a person's mental resources. Decisiveness, for example, belonged to the gall bladder, the capacity for calculated planning resided in the liver, craftiness belonged to the kidneys, and the sense of taste to the spleen.[20] Accounts of the heart in China offer little hint of the commanding dominance invested in the Greek *hegemonikon*. In the dynamics of the five phases, the heart conquered the lungs, but the heart in turn tended to be overpowered by the kidneys, the kidneys by the spleen, the spleen by the liver, and the liver by the lungs. Power circulated. No one *zang* lorded over all the others.

Read in isolation, the *Suwen*'s assertion that "The heart governs the *mo*" (*xin zhu mo*) may appear to contradict my thesis about blood and breath circulating without a ruling source. "The heart governs the *mo*" conjures up the image of a pumping heart and the pulsing arteries. The remarks that follow this declaration, however, indicate ties of another sort.

Yes, the heart governs the *mo*; but in the same way that the lungs govern the skin, the spleen governs the flesh, the liver governs the sinews, the kidneys govern the bones.[21] Considered carefully and as a whole, this list imparts a critical insight: the Chinese conception of the body differed from the body envisioned by Greek anatomy not just by the multiplicity and equality of governing sources, but also, and more profoundly, by an alternative conception of governance.

Block an artery, and the pulse disappears. Cut a nerve, and an arm falls limp. The effects are direct and immediate. It was through trials and observations of this kind that Galen demonstrated the heart's rule over the arteries and the brain's control of the muscles. And it is such connections that furnished the principal evidence for how the study of anatomical structure illuminates living function.

Governance (*zhu*) in Chinese medicine bound together parts in a rather different way. A weakening of the spleen may result in emaciation, and injury to the lungs may coarsen the skin, but there is an elusive indirectness to these effects that makes them quite unlike the paralysis caused by severing a nerve. Before the cause becomes fully manifest in the effect, days, months, even years may pass. We are dealing with connections spanning not just distant parts, but distant times. We are dealing with ties invisible to dissection.

What sort of ties were these? How did Chinese doctors conceive the structure of *zhu* governance? No story in Chinese medical history has been as often retold as that of Duke Huan's encounter with the legendary physician Bian Que:

> Bian Que passed through the state of Qi. The Duke of Qi invited him to be his guest. But when he was received by the Duke, Bian Que warned, "My Lord has a disease which lies in the pores. If it is not treated, it will sink deeper."

Duke Huan replied, "I am not sick."

Bian Que left. Duke Huan remarked to his attendants, "Physicians are greedy. They want to take credit for curing people who aren't even sick."

Five days later, Bian Que was received again. He warned the Duke, "My Lord has a disease which lies in the blood vessels. If it is not treated, I fear it will sink deeper."

The Duke replied, "I am not sick."

Bian Que left. The Duke was displeased. Five days later, Bian Que was received again. He urged the Duke, "My Lord has a disease which lies in the stomach and intestines. If it is not treated, it will sink deeper."

Duke Huan did not respond.

Bian Que left. The Duke was displeased. Five days later, Bian Que was received again. Gazing at Duke Huan from a distance, he retreated and rushed rapidly away. The Duke sent a man to ask Bian Que about the reasons for his behavior. Bian Que explained, "When the disease lies in the pores, it can be treated by poultices. When it lies in the blood vessels, it can be treated with needles. When it lies in the stomach and intestines, it can be treated with medicines. But when the disease lies in the bone marrow, not even the God of Life can do anything about it. The Duke's disease now lies in the bone marrow, and for this reason I have no more advice."

Five days later, the duke felt ill. Someone was sent to summon Bian Que, but he had already run away. Duke Huan subsequently died.[22]

Histories of Chinese medicine usually relate this anecdote, with varying degrees of critical distance, as a hagiographic testimonial to Bian Que's astonishing acumen; we could also read it plausibly, and more interestingly, as a cautionary tale about the limits of medicine as science, about how even divine insight is defeated by distrust. In the event, our concern is with its account of how a person gets sicker.

Ignorance and carelessness can aggravate a malady, a light sickness can become a grave affliction. Such language subtly associates pathology with intuitions of heaviness, *gravitas*, as if the advance of a illness were a process of the body becoming increasingly burdened, weighed down. By contrast, Bian Que's analysis of Duke Huan's demise appeals instead to a sense of spatial layering — to a conception of the body structured by the logic of depth and a theory of sickness understood as the progressive penetration of poisons. Breaching first the skin and pores, a disease sinks steadily, relentlessly inward — into the conduits, the sinews, the flesh, into the viscera, into the marrow of the bones. When it still hovers near the pores it can be expelled by poultices, say, or acupuncture; as it burrows deeper, medicines must be ingested; until eventually the disease infiltrates the marrow, where no cures can reach.

By what process do imperceptible disorders evolve into deadly diseases? Although the interpretation sketched above appears in Sima Qian's biography of Bian Que — that is, in a historical narrative rather than in a technical treatise — it captures the schematic essence of what we find in the medical classics as well. The *Neijing* portrays sicknesses arising and unfolding in a great variety of patterns — including spreading outward, sometimes, from the inner viscera; yet amid this diversity we find certain recurring themes, exemplary paradigms which physicians knew couldn't explain all afflictions, but which nonetheless summarized their innermost sense of what sickness was all about. Of these paradigms the most powerful and influential was that which imagined noxious breaths from without infiltrating into the layered space of the body.

"Harmful winds come upon one as swiftly as the wind and

rain," the *Suwen* asserts, and "the most skillful healer treats the surface hairs (*pimao*)." Winds are "the beginning of the hundred diseases," and those doctors are best who disperse them before they sweep inward. "The healer next in skill treats the subcutaneous tissues (*jifu*); the healer next in skill after that treats the sinews and vessels; the healer next in skill after that treats the six hollow viscera; the healer next in skill after that treats the five solid viscera. When one treats the five solid viscera, one is treating someone who is already half dead, only half alive...."[23] Both the skill of healers and the seriousness of diseases could thus be mapped in space, measured by the layers separating the fine hairs at the body surface from the solid viscera deep inside.

Right after this ranking of healers the *Suwen* proffers the synopsis of palpation quoted in chapter 1: "In palpating the *chi* and the *cun*, one checks whether the *mo* is floating or sunken, slippery and rough, and knows the origin of the disease."[24]

The claims of slipperiness and roughness, we learned before, mirrored the primacy of flow in the imagination of the *mo*. Now we can appreciate the special import of the floating and the sunken. If you place your fingers lightly and feel an abundance, but the *mo* disappears as the fingers press harder, that *mo* is called floating; if, on the contrary, you sense nothing with a light touch, but discover abundance upon pressing deeper, that is a sunken *mo*. This pair communicates the nature of a sickness, *Lingshu* treatise 59 explains: the floating and the sunken correspond, respectively, to superficial and deep afflictions.[25] *Suwen* treatise 18 likewise asserts: a sunken, hard *mo* means that the disease lies inside; a floating, swelling *mo* indicates harmful breaths besieging the surface — the skin, the pores, the sinews.[26]

Not that the two always signaled sickness. In spring, for instance, it was natural that the *mo* should float, as vital energies

165

radiated outward; and in winter the *mo* normally sank as the blood and *qi* retreated inward. The floating *mo* is yang, and the sunken *mo* is yin, says *Nanjing* 4. The opposition of floating versus sunken ranked as perhaps the most fundamental distinction in *qiemo*, and this because in Chinese medicine all changes in the body, physiological as well as pathological, were governed by the logic of depth.

Floating and sunken were actually invoked in two separate senses. Besides specifying certain *qualities* in the *mo*, the pair also named fixed *sites* of palpation. Recall: *cunkou* diagnosis trisected the wrist horizontally into the *cun*, *guan*, and *chi*, but each of these in turn was also split vertically into the floating and sunken *positions*. This is how doctors diagnosed six viscera at each wrist. At the floating position, feeling the *mo* with minimal pressure, they divined the condition of the hollow *fu*, the yang organs; at the sunken position, pressing down harder, they inquired into the *zang*, the solid yin viscera governing the *fu*.

Nanjing 5 proposed further vertical refinements. Press on the *mo* lightly, with the weight of three beans, and you learn the state of the skin and the pores and of the *zang* that governed them, namely, the lungs; press a bit harder, with the pressure of six beans, you test the condition of the blood vessels and their governing *zang*, the heart; a third level corresponds to the flesh and spleen, a fourth level to the tendons and liver, and the deepest level, felt with the pressure of fifteen beans, reveals the state of the bones and their principal *zang*, the kidneys.[27]

Galen lingered on the flawless fit between form and function, marveling at how the shape of each organ perfectly expressed its use. In China, morphology inspired no comparable enthusiasms. Shape mattered far less than place: the functional structure of the human body was ordered first and foremost by the polarity opposing the body surface (*biao*) to its inner core (*li*).

166

So the enigma of visual knowledge in Chinese medicine can be put thus: How does one contemplate a body organized by depth?

The solution of Chinese doctors was to gaze upon the surface. To the anatomical eye, the skin is an occluding screen, blocking insight into underlying forms, and a body without forms is but uninformative matter, darkly inscrutable. But in China the skin shone as the site of privileged revelations. For there, at the surface, doctors contemplated a person's *se* — as in *wuse*, the five colors. If Hellenistic dissectors scrutinized the functional meaning of organic shape, healers in Han-dynasty China peered into the profound significance of hue.

The Object of the Gaze

Each sense has objects that are proper to it, which define its role in diagnosis. The fingers, for instance, feel the texture of the skin, the warmth and consistency of the flesh, the flow of the *mo*. The nose smells the patient's body and excretions. The ears hear voice pitch, groans, reports of pain and malaise. As for the eyes, they observe many things — physique, gait, posture, edemas, skin eruptions. But mainly, seeing in Chinese medicine entailed gazing upon color (*wangse*). The contemplation of colors defined, theoretically, the use and rationale of sight; and in practice, too, it was colors that commanded the most intense and searching scrutiny.

Why? Were someone to ask us what a doctor must eye, the word "color" likely wouldn't spring immediately to mind. "Smells" seems a natural reply to "What should the nose sniff?," and we readily accept "Sounds" as an answer to "What should the ears hear?" But the distillation of sight to the perception of color catches us off guard.

Not that there is anything odd about an interest in hue. A face tinged with yellow or red, the *Neijing* suggests, indicates fever; white means cold; green and black, pain.[28] In fevers of the liver, redness first appears on the left cheek; in fevers of the lung, on the right cheek; in cardiac fevers, on the forehead.[29] We may distrust some of these interpretations, but the intuition behind them is certainly familiar. We, too, read sickness in the pallor, or feverish flush, or jaundice of the faces around us.

Rather, what perplexes is that seeing should be *equated with* perceiving *se*, and that perceiving *se* should reign over other forms of knowing. Colors may reveal pain and fever and cold, but these are broad problems with countless nuances and causes, and they can all be diagnosed in other ways. The possibility of detecting them, by itself, could hardly justify the privileging of *se*.

And, indeed, classical medical theory advanced a second, more general rationale. It taught that the microcosmic body, like the greater macrocosm, was ruled by the interactions between the *wuxing*, or five phases (wood, fire, earth, metal, and water), and that the waxing and waning of these *wuxing* manifested itself in, among other things, the flourishing and fading of the *wuse* — the five colors, green, red, yellow, white, and black. Color thus had cosmic significance.

From the hue tinging the face, doctors could know the phase that ruled the illness. A florid countenance bespoke ascendant fire; a visage with yellowish tints, the waxing of earth.[30] Actual diagnosis naturally became more involved, as doctors balanced nuances of shade, differences in when and where various hues appeared, and the testimony of other senses.[31] But the principle was elementary: healers eyed the five colors as manifestations of the fivefold forces of cosmic change.

Already established in the Han classics of medicine, this perception of color subsequently defined the analytical framework of all postclassical commentary on visual knowledge. It persists even today as the standard rationale recited by textbooks of traditional medicine to explain the meaning of gazing upon *se*.

In Qin and Han times, physicians weren't alone in perceiving great portents in hue, and the five-phase view of color carried special conviction. For political theorists, the five colors symbolized the rise and fall of dynasties. White was the color of the Shang dynasty; red, the hue of the succeeding Zhou. The latter's conquest of the former was presaged, legend had it, by the capture of a white fish and the appearance of a beam of light, which transformed itself into a bright red crow.[32] The first Qin emperor linked the fortunes of his own dynasty with the water that conquers red (*Zhou*) fire, and ordered black (water's chromatic correlate) for the official banners and ceremonial dress of his court.[33]

Nor were the implications of hue confined to succession in time. Color also reflected the partition of space, the dynamics of the four quarters. Sima Qian (145–90 B.C.E.) records a ritual in which the emperor erected a five-colored mound as an altar to the spirits of the land. The mound was made of green soil on the east, red soil on the south, white soil on the west, black soil on the north, and covered on top with yellow soil—the last representing the imperial center. When a prince was enfeoffed with land to the east, he received some of the green soil; a prince whose fief lay in the south received red soil; a prince whose fief lay in the west received white soil; and a prince whose fief lay in the north received black soil. Each then would take this soil to his fief and build an altar around it, covering it with the yellow earth that he would also receive.[34]

Color symbolized power. Chromatic consciousness suffused Han political culture and was aggressively displayed in court banners and ritual utensils, in clothing and architectural design. That the cosmic resonance of the five colors heightened medical consciousness of hues scarcely brooks doubt.

Still, it cannot entirely explain the fixation on *se*. Turning to Chinese beliefs about the role and nature of sight, we find that two stubborn puzzles remain.

One concerns the mystique of the gaze. After all, associations with cosmic rhythms weren't unique to sight. Nothing in five-phase analysis promoted the eyes as more discerning than the ears or the nose, or made the five colors more oracular than the five sounds or five smells. If sight crowned a hierarchy of ways of knowing, if to gaze and know was divine, the reason had to lie elsewhere than what the *wuse* might teach about the *wuxing*.

A skeptic could argue, to be sure, that this hierarchy expressed more a theoretical ideal than the reality of practice. In the insightful diagnosis that so impressed the Emperor He, remember, Guo Yu wasn't allowed to see anything at all, but had to grasp the truth just by feeling two wrists thrust through curtain openings. After the discovery of the *mo*, we hear few echoes of Bian Que's power to see through walls.

Yet even if the primacy of sight was merely an ideal, it still needs explaining *as* an ideal. Moreover, the canonical classics of Chinese medicine leave no doubt that even after the ascendance of *qiemo*, sight retained special claims. To the five sounds, five smells, and five tastes, the *Neijing* and *Nanjing* generally give only brief, perfunctory treatment. One gets the impression, sometimes, that they are mentioned simply as gestures toward comprehensiveness. Not so with sight. "[Knowledge of] *se* and the *mo*," *Suwen* treatise 13 asserts, "are what the ancient sage-kings prized, and what the early masters transmitted." To know *se* and the *mo* was to know the essential, and it was through these two that the sages of the golden past attained divine clarity.[35] "The physician who can combine the *mo* and *se*," proclaims *Suwen* treatise 10, "achieves perfection."[36] *Qiemo* may eventually have become the primary and most trusted means of diagnosis, but inspection of *se* always remained its necessary complement.[37]

Somehow, the two were inseparable: reliable assessment of the *mo* required weighing ocular evidence, and vice versa. "*Se* corresponds to the yang, and the *mo* to the yin."[38] If the indications of color and the *mo* matched each other — if, for example, both indicated a wood ailment — then the patient would live; if they diverged, if one signaled wood and the other metal, the patient would die.[39] The ear, nose, and tongue might add supplemental hints, but the real crux of judgment lay in the dialectic of hand and eye. "Those skilled in diagnosis scrutinize *se* and palpate the *mo*."[40] For all the importance of palpation, one couldn't truly know the body without knowing *se*.[41]

The correspondence between the five colors and the five phases, however, doesn't tell us why.

A second puzzle concerns the fact that the focus on *se* wasn't particular to medicine.

> The way the mouth is disposed toward tastes, the eye toward colors (*se*), the ear toward sounds, the nose toward smells, and the four limbs toward ease is human nature....[42]

Mencius here echoes the standard partition of the senses in ancient China: color is to the eye what taste is to the mouth and sound to the ear.[43] Color is not *one* object of sight, any more than smell is one object of olfaction; it is *the* object of sight, the yearning toward which defines the eye's very nature. The enigma of *se*, therefore, doesn't merely concern the medical diagnosis of colors. Just as Greek study of anatomical structures was rooted in a broader philosophical discourse on forms, so the contemplation of *se* engaged commitments that reached well beyond healing.

But what commitments? What bound the human eye, and not just the diagnostic gaze, to *se*? Besides broadening the scope of our problem, Mencius's remarks hint again at the incompleteness of any account of *se* confined to the five colors. Mencius (371–289? B.C.E.) was born more than a century before the compilation of the *Lüshi chunqiu* (240 B.C.E.), which was the first work systematically to apply five-phase analysis to a theory of cosmic correspondences. To be sure, much remains uncertain about the early history of five-phase thinking, and we can find groupings of things into sets of five — and indeed, the phrases *wuxing* and *wuse* — in texts presumably antedating or contemporary with Mencius.[44] Yet in the *Mencius* itself, the phrase *wuse* doesn't appear even once, and this despite the fact that the term *se* appears some two dozen times. More tellingly still, neither in the references to the five colors prior to the *Lüshi chunqiu*, nor in Mencius's comments on color, do we find any suggestion that the eye fixes on colors *because* there are five colors or *because* of a connection between color and cosmic change. Five-phase analysis alone, in sum, can't account for the marriage of sight and *se*.

The Meanings of Se

Yet perhaps the attachment to color isn't so odd. Aristotle, too, in his treatise on the soul, asserts that the object of sight is "the visible" (*to horaton*) and then elaborates, "The visible is color."[45] And if we count white and black as colors, as the Chinese certainly did, we too must acknowledge the elementary character of hue: without shades of light and dark we would be unable even to discern shapes. We would see nothing at all.

Colors often glow, furthermore, with mystical associations. In their burial rituals, the *Liji* tells us, the people of Yin (Shang) times "treasured [the color] white."[46] The important Shang ritual known as the *liao* sacrifice called specifically for the burning of a white dog; and inscriptional references in other contexts to white cows, white horses, white pigs, and white deer all underline the symbolic resonance of white in Shang culture.[47] Long before their interpretation was systematized and rationalized by five-phase theorists, in other words, colors signified.

Neither of these considerations, however, solve our puzzle, and this most immediately because they aren't explicitly acknowledged. When Mencius and others yoked the eye to *se*, they appealed neither to the symbolism of hues, nor to the perceptual priority of shades over forms. Then there is this decisive limitation: all the reasons for fixing on color can never fully elucidate the equation of seeing with seeing *se*, because seeing *se* wasn't just a matter of perceiving colors. Although the term *se* appears fairly commonly in pre-Han writings, more often than not it didn't designate hue — at least not simply and directly.

The related compound *yanse* is instructive here. In modern Mandarin, *yanse* is the standard word for color. To learn the hue of a friend's new Toyota, you ask, "What is its *yanse*?" But *yanse* is an ancient term and figures already in the *Analects* — though for Confucius it had a rather different sense: "Confucius said, 'When in attendance at a gentleman one is liable to three errors. To speak before being spoken to by the gentleman is rash; not to speak when spoken to by him is to be evasive; to speak without observing the expression on his face (*yanse*) is to be blind.'"[48] *Yanse* thus meant not color but facial expression. This passage is typical of classical usage: nowhere in early Chinese writings does *yanse* refer to the abstract idea of hue. Originally, it spoke exclusively of the look on a person's face.

The character *yan* designates the face, or more precisely, the forehead, and from this one might suppose that *se* by itself meant something like look or appearance. And indeed, in postclassical Buddhist usage *se* named the realm of phenomenal appearance, as opposed to noumenal emptiness (*kong*). Were this its sense in antiquity the identification of seeing with seeing *se* would be trivial, for *se* would encompass all sense perception.

However, in pre-Buddhist writings the term wasn't metaphysical. Most often, *se* evoked not appearance in general, but specifically the appearance of the face. Whenever Confucius crossed the station of his lord, "his face suddenly changed expression (*se*), his step became brisk, and his words more laconic.... When he had come out and descended the first step, he relaxed his expression (*yanse*) and no longer seemed tense."[49] In this passage, facial expression is first called *se*, and then *yanse*, but the two are clearly synonymous. In late Zhou and Warring States usage, mien, not hue, was *se*'s usual sense.

Mencius thus observes the hungry air (*jise*) of the people under a tyrant,[50] and the joyful expression (*xise*) of a people blessed with a generous king;[51] and Zhuangzi spots the woeful mien (*youse*) of those who have yet to awaken to the Way.[52] Eventually, with the rise of five-color/five-phase analysis, the association of *se* and color becomes fairly common. Even so, the Han dynasty *Shuowen*, the earliest Chinese dictionary, defines *se* as "the spirit (*qi*) [that appears in] the forehead"; and much later, the Qing commentator Duan Yucai would still explain, "*Yan* refers to the space between the eyebrows. The mind appears in the spirit (*qi*), and the spirit appears in the forehead. This is what is called *se*." The modern *Cihai*, in fact, still lists "spirit of the face" (*yanqi*) as *se*'s first meaning, citing Duan's comments for support. Color appears as the second sense.

This suggests one explanation (I shall later advance another) for why the Chinese spoke of *gazing* upon *se*. Current summaries of traditional medicine frequently explain diagnostic inspection as if it were a straightforward mechanical task: to learn which of the five phases is ascendant one simply looks at the hue on the patient's face. Yet *wang*, to gaze — the standard verb for inspecting *se* — intimates a subtler art.

Early inscriptions represent *wang* by a graph for the eye combined with a picture of someone stretching forward (𝑘). The mature version of the character (望) shows a person leaning forward to catch a glimpse of the distant moon. Both forms reflect the etymology of the term: *wang*, to gaze, was cognate with *wang*, to be absent, and *mang*, to be obscure.[53] In other words, *wang* (to gaze) expressed the effort to see what can be perceived only darkly, or in the distance. Seeing *se* somehow involved a straining of the eyes, the reach toward something absent or obscure.

Interpreting *se* as countenance illuminates one source of this sense of straining. For what do we see when we perceive a look? Raised eyebrows, a glimmer in the eyes, pursed lips, the lack or flush of color. All these doubtless form part of what we take in. But mostly, we don't attend to them separately and consciously, any more than we read a book letter by letter. Rather, what we see, or think we see — it is often difficult truly to be sure — are hesitation or impatience, despair or longing, shiftiness or candor. That is, we gaze upon attitudes and inclinations, which are distinctly visible, yet hard to see distinctly.

The habit of gazing upon *se* likely began in this way. Medical study of facial hues grew out of a long fascination with facial expressions. The puzzle of Chinese seeing is only partly about color. It is also about reading faces.

Perceptual Desires

Our concern is with what the Chinese sought to learn from faces — that is, with *se* as an object of knowledge. But no discussion of *se* can ignore how it also stirred desire.

Look again at the passage from Mencius: "The way the mouth is disposed toward tastes, the eye toward colors (*se*), the ear toward sounds, the nose toward smells, and the four limbs toward ease is human nature...."

Mentioning limbs alongside the eyes, nose, and mouth may seem incongruous. The eyes, nose, and mouth are perceptual organs, after all, whereas the limbs are not. Nonetheless, the relationship between the limbs and ease parallels that between the senses and their objects in one telling respect: both are relationships of desire. Colors, smells, and tastes are not just what the eyes, the nose, and mouth perceive, not just objects of sensory knowledge. They are targets of sensual yearning. Zhuangzi puts it bluntly: "Such are human feelings: the eye yearns to see colors (se), the ear to hear sounds, the mouth to savor tastes."[54]

And the craving for se is strongest. "I have yet to meet the man," Confucius observes, "who is as fond of virtue as he is of beauty (se)."[55] Human nature consists in the appetite for food and sex (se), Gaozi suggests.[56] After facial expression, these are the most common senses of se: beauty and the desires that it arouses.

Se makes a woman proud, but the favors and affections it fosters wilt as it fades.[57] A passion for se, haose, is a weakness of nearly all flawed rulers; resistance to its seductions, a mark of superior character.[58] From the earliest chronicles, se's fatal lure looms large in Chinese historiography as the downfall of many a state. Se identified lust as visual craving.

Implicit in the general equation of seeing with seeing se, then, was an element of natural attraction. Se wasn't just what the eyes could or should perceive, but what they *wanted* to see.

Was this desire related in any way to the preoccupation with se in medicine? *Haose* and *wangse*, visual lust and the diagnostic gaze. At first blush, the two seem completely unrelated, opposites even. *Haose* conjured up a se of dazzling allure, while the se of *wangse* was fleeting and elusive. Moralists enjoined people to turn away from the former, while doctors were encouraged to study the latter intently. Still, they were both called *se* — which surely isn't coincidence.

Let us look deeper into what appears on the face.

Se *as Expression*

Faces reveal much about the people around us, but reading them requires finesse.

Expressions are at best translucent, and people can dissimulate. The *Shujing*, one of the earliest Chinese texts, already warns against selecting officers on the basis of cunning words and ingratiating faces (*qiaoyan lingse*);[59] and Confucius likewise cautions that "a man of cunning words and ingratiating face is rarely benevolent."[60] More than once in the *Analects* we find the Master voicing his wariness of the chasm between facades of benevolence, friendliness, and bravery, and a person's real disposition.[61] Of course, such warnings weren't intended so much to deny the face's truth as to underline the need for insight. "If a king knows people," the *Shujing* says, "why should he fear cunning words and ingratiating faces?"[62]

Perspicacious observers can see through pretense and espy even silent thoughts, hidden plans. Duke Huan of Qi once plotted with his minister Guan Zhong to attack Lu. Mysteriously, even before they had announced their plans, word of the impending expedition had spread. "There must be a remarkable sage in the land," Guan Zhong exclaimed. Only a sage could have fathomed unspoken designs. Suspecting a certain Dongguo Ya, he summoned him and asked,

"Were you the one who announced the attack on Lu?"
"Indeed."
"I said nothing about attacking Lu. How did you know?"

Responded Dongguo Ya: it was a simple matter of observing Guan Zhong's face (*se*). Over time, Dongguo Ya had learned to see when Guan Zhong was joyful, or pensive, or riled for battle. By reading the minister's expression in the context of current politics, he had divined what was in store.[63]

Wang Chong (27–100), who recounts this incident, then goes on to relate another tale about how the sharp-eyed Chunyu Kun astonished King Hui of Liang by reading the king's wandering thoughts. And he sums up, "The intention was inside the breast, hidden and invisible, but Kun was able to know it." How? "He contemplated the face to peer into the mind" (*guanse yi kuixin*).[64]

The amazement aroused by such access to secrets goes far toward clarifying the mystique surrounding sight. Even in Wang Chong's account of events, the acuity of the two sages is impressive. But Wang was an exception in his time, a staunch rationalist who sought to refute widespread belief in supernatural prophecy. His interpretation of the feats of Dongguo Ya and Chunyu Kun argued against a popular tradition that idolized these men as diviners — *seers* who, like Bian Que, could behold what lay concealed inside bodies, in minds, in time.

Here was another reason for speaking of "gazing" upon color: the close association of seeing and divining. Physicians gazed at a patient's look (*wangse*) and predicted the course of illness, much as another class of diviners gazed at the air (*wangqi*) and prophesied the fate of armies and states.[65] *Wangqi* was a mantic art that became especially popular in the Qin and Western Han dynasties, around the same time that medicine was beginning to coalesce into its classical form.[66] Its premise was that shifts in climate, in political fortunes, and above all in the momentum of battles appeared first as subtle changes in the atmosphere.[67]

When the clouds floating above an army take the shape of a beast, *wangqi* experts taught, then the army will triumph. Wispy, clear white clouds signal a ruthless leader with fearful troops. Greenish white clouds that dip low presage victory. Clouds reddish in the front and rising, warn that the battle cannot be won. In some regions the atmosphere is white, in others red, in yet others the lower sky is black and the upper air is blue. "One divines by matching the clouds and the five colors."[68]

On his accession to the throne (59 B.C.E.), Emperor Ming of the Han dynasty climbed atop the observation platform of the Heavenly Altar and "gazed into the clouds" to discern the shifting ethers that would influence his reign.[69] Gazing at *qi* entailed scrutinizing distant clouds and air to peer into the obscurity of things to come.

Contemplating *se* in medicine was remarkably similar. In both *wangse* and *wangqi* the seer strained to detect the first, most ethereal manifestations of change. When a particularly powerful pathogen attacks the body, the *Lingshu* relates, "the patient shivers and trembles and moves the body." The illness appears in violent shaking that no one can miss. But when the pathogen is less virulent, the symptoms are initially much subtler: "The illness can first be seen in the face (*se*), even though it may not appear in the body. It seems to be there, but not there; it seems to exist, yet not exist; it seems to be visible, and yet invisible. No one can describe it."[70]

Wang er zhi zhi — to gaze and know things, the pinnacle of medical acumen — was thus to know things before they had taken form, to grasp "what is there and yet not there." As an illness becomes more serious, its corresponding color intensifies. If the color fades "like clouds completely dispersing (*yun chesan*)," the illness will soon pass. One observes whether the color is superficial or sunken to know the depth of the illness, whether the color is dispersed or concentrated to know the proximity of crises. "By concentrating the mind in this way, one can know [changes]

179

past and present."[71] Before an illness crystallizes in the body, it announces itself in the face, in an altered air.

Western commentaries on Chinese medicine and philosophy frequently stress the holistic unity of the Chinese body/self. For a predictable reason: viewed against the dualisms that have so forcefully framed Western readings of the human condition — the radical oppositions of divine spirit and corrupt flesh, of immaterial mind and material body — the absence of such polarities leaps out as *the* critical difference. But the surprise at not finding these dichotomies in Chinese thought has often induced the neglect of distinctions that the Chinese did make. One such distinction is that between form and face — or, to be exact, between *xing* and *se*. *Xing* and *se* (*xingse*), Mencius tells us, are our natural endowment.[72]

We can glean a general sense of the distinction from some closely parallel phrases — *xingshen* (form and spirit), *xingsheng* (form and vitality), *xingqi* (form and breath). The intuition voiced by these phrases, that of humans beings as a composite of form and something else, bears an unmistakable family resemblance to the bifurcation of body and soul. With a significant difference, though: what separated *se* from *xing* wasn't ontological essence, but degrees of perspicuity.

As the *Lingshu* passage suggests, there are aspects and phenomena — gross morphology, the shaking of the limbs and trunk — that one can't miss. Then there is the more ethereal, more volatile *se*, aspects of a person which are still visible but are fleeting and dim, which "seem to be there but not there, seem to exist and yet not exist."

Doctors treasured *se* because it signaled the faintest changes. Physique and physiognomy metamorphose over months and years; by the time an illness reshapes these, it has usually been long at work. Yet well before an illness emaciates and disfigures, it appears in fugitive and ineffable changes in look. The physician who gazes and knows, who truly sees *se*, perceives realities that remain invisible to others until much later.

Attention to *se* was also a moral duty. A person who has "gotten through" (*da*) and grasped the Way, according to Confucius, "is straight by nature and fond of what is right, *sensitive to other people's words and observant of the expression on their faces*, and always mindful of being modest" (italics added).[73]

"The expression on their faces" translates *se*. By ranking it alongside such cardinal virtues as rectitude, righteousness, and modesty, Confucius invested the observation of faces with a stature that we ourselves don't normally accord it. We can guess, though, why Confucius thought this way; the reason surely lay in his vision of moral development, which made cultivating the self inseparable from relating to others. To respond appropriately to people we must understand them. To understand them we must attend carefully to their words and faces.

Yet what is it exactly that we must understand in others? What do faces and words express? Recall the discussion of language in chapter 2. A familiar paradigm conceives words as symbols for intentions and ideas. In this model, to understand a word is to grasp the idea that the word represents. The Confucian stress on verbal sensitivity sprang from other assumptions. Think back to Mencius's explanation of "knowing words": "When words are extravagant, I know how the mind is fallen and sunk. When words are depraved, I know how the mind has departed from principle. When words are evasive, I know how the mind is at its wit's end."[74]

"Knowing words" thus had little to do with lucid definition or intelligence about particular terms. Rather, to know words was to hear the attitudes and states of mind from which words sprang. Sensitive listening was listening to the unintentional overtones of intentional speech.

A similar hermeneutic motivated the contemplation of faces. To the observant eye, *se* expressed even those inclinations that people wanted to conceal, even velleities of which they themselves were unaware. Thus when people "change expression" (*bianse*), or "make a face" (*zuose*), they are often described as doing so suddenly, spontaneously — *boran bianse, boran zuose, fenran zuose, furan zuose* — without premeditation, caught by surprise, seized by fury.[75] Such phrases testify to the easy transition from expression to hue. We could translate as well, "suddenly change color," or "suddenly color" — or more expansively, "blenched in shock," "flushed with rage," "blushed in shame."

In *se*, people show their true colors. When Confucius emerged from an official audience, he "manifested his *yanse*" — translators say, "he relaxed his expression" — letting down his guard, allowing his feelings to show through. In observing *se*, we observe the self.

Stunned and humiliated by the criticism of a sardonic gardener-sage, Zi Gong "lost his *se*":

> Dazed and rattled, he couldn't seem to pull himself together (*bu zi de*) and it was only after he had walked on for some thirty *li* that he began to recover.
>
> One of his disciples said, "Who was that man just now? Why did you change your expression and lose your color (*shi se*) like that, Master, so that it took you all day to get back to normal (*zhongri bu zi fan*)?"[76]

Bu zide translates more literally as, "couldn't regain self-possession"; and *zhongri bu zi fan* as "couldn't recover your self for the whole day." Loss of *se* entailed at once losing color and losing the self.

A moment ago, I contrasted the gradual, long-term character

of alterations in fleshly form (*xing*) to the ethereal volatility of *se*. But of course facial expressions don't change randomly, nor do they just mirror momentary provocations. They also express deliberate disciplines and settled habits of mind.

Chinese thinkers knew this well. *Se* claimed their attention not just as an object, something seen, but also as something to be subjectively cultivated. Though he denounced meretricious pretense, Confucius himself made mastery of demeanor central to the cultivation of self: "There are three things that the gentleman values most in the Way: to stay clear of violence by putting on a serious countenance, to come close to being trusted by setting a proper expression on his face, and to avoid being boorish and unreasonable by speaking in proper tones."[77]

Two of the three most valued virtues thus called for managing the face; the third concerned speech. Note again the linkage of *se* and words, and recall how the crux of speech lay not so much in the ideas explicitly opined, as in the *ciqi*, the implicit spirit of discourse. The expressiveness of the face was like the expressiveness of a person's tone of speech.

> Zi Xia asked about being filial. The Master said, "What is difficult to manage is the expression on one's face (*senan*). As for the young taking on the burden when there is work to be done or letting the old enjoy the wine and the food when these are available, that hardly deserves to be called filial."[78]

Taking on onerous chores, providing for elderly parents — these are things that filial children must do; but they don't suffice to make one filial. Filial duties must be performed with the proper face. And therein lies the challenge. Just like in the performance of rites: "Unless a man has the spirit of the rites, in being respectful he will wear himself out, in being careful he will become timid."[79] Anyone can utter certain words, walk, clasp their hands, bow. They are easy: one decides to do them, and does them. But tone of voice, bearing, facial expression, the precise spirit of the ritual — these are another matter. Like walking and bowing, they are subject to the will, but one's control over them is less consistent, more tenuous and indirect. They need patient cultivation over time, repeated practice.

Se thus expressed the years of lived life, sometimes in the most concrete sense. Zhuangzi speaks for instance of a seventy-year-old sage whose complexion (*se*) was that of a young babe.[80] The biography of Hua Tuo marvels at how the arts of rejuvenation gave him the countenance (*se*) of youth even in old age.[81] In both cases, *se* translates either as complexion or face, and probably encompasses both. Part of what we observe in judging age is facial expression — whether someone looks experienced or untested, life-weary or callow. But we also note the color, softness, and sheen of the skin. As an indicator of age or health *se* was thus synonymous with *seli*, where *li* referred to the pores of the skin, and *seze*, where *ze* evoked the skin's luster. *Seli* and *seze* thus evoked skin hue and texture, the life manifest on the surface. Hua Tuo and Zhuangzi's sage were old in years, but *looked* young. This is another aspect of people's looks, whether they appear youthful or decrepit.

We find an interesting parallel to *se* in the Homeric notion of *chrōs*. For *chrōs*, too, pointed toward the expressively tinged face. The divide between the cowardly and the brave, the captain of the Cretans observes, is clear: "The color [of a coward] is ever-changing" (*trepetai chrōs allydis allē*; Fitzgerald translates, "This one's face goes greener by the minute"), whereas "The color [of the brave one] never changes." But *chrōs* was also the vital body. It refers, for example, to the body of Patrocles, preserved by nectar and ambrosia, or the body of Achilles, which must (or so Agenor thinks), like that of all mortals, be vulnerable to bronze spears. Hector's body/flesh (*chrōs*), despite being subject to desecrations, remains strangely preserved.[82] The subsequent rise of humoral analysis in Greek medicine doubtless owed something to this vision of body as flesh tinged with life.

The predominance of yellow or black bile, phlegm or blood appeared in facial hues of yellow or black, or white or red. Thus Greek physicians, too, took account of color in their diagnoses, and Galen could even identify sight with the apprehension of chromatic change.[83] The second-century treatise on physiognomy by Polemo included several chapters on the interpretation of complexions.[84] Still, *se* in Chinese medicine engaged an intensity of interest and had a range of significance unmatched by colors in Greek medicine.

Moreover, Chinese colors weren't humoral. The *Lingshu* remarks that poor circulation causes loss of luster in the face and hair; and this is as close as the Chinese classics come to a humoral account.[85] Which raises an intriguing question: If not as a mix of colored fluids, how did Chinese physicians imagine the hue tinging the face? Why *does* the face have color?

The Flowering Spirit

I have thus far spoken loosely of *se*'s expressiveness — of faces mirroring feelings and inclinations, of hues displaying the waxing and waning of the five-phases within a person. To conclude, I should like to inquire into precisely *how se* was related to what it expressed.

The relationship between a person and a person's look is surely not the same as that between the decision to start walking and the contraction of the relevant muscles. Showing a look involves more than just a decision; one can try to look filial, but effort alone hardly insures success. Nor is the relationship between *se* and what it expresses like that between the artifacts of Plato's craftsman and the ideas of which these artifacts are the material realization. It isn't a matter of foresightful design.

Volition and intention can play a part, of course. People sometimes strive for a certain look, and this effort influences how, indeed, they look. To command respect and obedience among his followers, the duke of Bi rectified the expression on his face (*zhengse*); Kong Fu set a proper expression on his face and presented himself at court;[86] the *Analects* hearken repeatedly to the expressions assumed by the Master. But looks that are truly commanding, or reverent, or benevolent — as opposed to mere facades of authority, or reverence, or benevolence — can't be summoned anytime, by anyone who might will them. Something more is needed.

Further, we've noted that often it is precisely in one's unguarded moments that *se* expresses most, despite oneself. The limited role of will and purposive design holds all the more in the case of *se* as it expresses age or health. One's color, the luster and elasticity of the skin, and a look of youthfulness and vitality or the absence thereof — all these express the will only indirectly, if at all, as the sum of countless decisions and indecisions spanning months and years.

How then should we imagine *se*'s expressiveness? More to the point, how was this expressiveness conceived in ancient China?

The recurrent imagery of flowering offers a hint. "Color," the *Suwen* declares, "is the flower (or flowering) of the spirit (*sezhe, qi zhi hua ye*)." "The heart gathers together the essences of the five zang.... The flowering visage (*huase*), is their bloom." And again, "The heart unites the *mo*, and it flowers in the face (*qi rong se ye*)."[87]

Botanical metaphors appear so ubiquitously in Chinese writings that we are apt to take such remarks for granted. Yet in them

186

we may discover one answer to our earlier query about the relationship between the various viscera and the parts that each governs. And that answer is: it is just like in plants. Governing viscera and governed parts, the vital inner core and the expressive surface — all these are related in the same way that roots and stem are related to the leaves and blossoms.

When the spleen ceases to nourish, the flesh becomes soft and the tongue wilts (*wei*); when the kidneys cease to nourish, the bones become desiccated (*ku*).[88] Similarly, the correspondence between *qi* on the one hand, and *se* and *mo* on the other, is like that between trunk and branch, roots and leaves (*benmo genye*).[89] According to the *Nanjing*, the source of vital breath (*shengqi*) serves as the body's stem and roots. When the roots are severed, the branches and leaves wither.[90] The *Shanghanlun* explains, "When the protective *qi* declines, then the face becomes yellow; when the nourishing *qi* declines, the face becomes green. The nourishing *qi* forms the root; the protective *qi*, the leaves. When both are feeble, then the roots and leaves become withered and desiccated."[91]

Such passages abound. Of all the metaphors deployed in imagining the body, none figured as centrally as the metaphor of plant growth and development.[92] The flowering face can be seen as one instance of this recurring trope.

I should say: an especially revealing instance. For it suggests that the botanical vision of the body was a vision in the literal, as well as figurative sense. Physicians didn't merely speak of *se* as flower, but *saw* it as such. They scrutinized the face in much the same way that a gardener eyes the flourishing or decline of his plants.

Obvious signs of a plant in faltering health include limpness, shriveling, and desiccation, and Chinese doctors described the sickly body in exactly the same terms. But the subtlest and most revealing index of vitality appears in the color and luster of the blossoms. When I lived in Atlanta, my neighbor was a devoted gardener, while I neglected my yard. Each spring, the difference was embarrassingly apparent: my neighbor's azaleas blazed with a rich brilliance of color that bespoke the fertilized soil on which they had been painstakingly nourished. My own azaleas (planted, in any case, by a previous owner) had the recriminatingly pale hues of plants left to scrounge in Georgia clay. The leaves of my neighbor's plants literally shone with lustrous life. Mine looked sadly dull and drab.

Tellingly, the contemplation of the face in Chinese medicine called for kindred observations. Ultimately, the most vital distinctions turned less on bald differences in color — seeing white, say, where pink would have been the healthier — than on the contrast between lustrous and lackluster shades of the same hue. The glistening white, and red, and black, of pig's fat, the cock's mane, and crow feathers all portended recovery. The dull white, red, and black of dried bones, coagulated blood, and soot signaled death.[93]

Earlier we noted a curious duality in *se*. Besides the *se* of *wangse*, there was also the *se* that inspired yearning. In various contexts, the term is best translated as "beauty" or "sexual attractiveness." "As for those who traffic in *se*," moralizes the *Zhanguoce*, "the blossoms will fall and affections will change." The *Shiji* reminds those "who use *se* to manipulate others": when *se* fades, affection wilts.[94] Though beauty and passion bloom radiant, like blossoms, sooner or later they fade and go limp. These are commonplaces. Yet read attentively, they hint at the deeper springs of desire.

Why should *se* — color, facial expression, air — also mean beauty and sexual attractiveness? The analogy to plants suggests that one aspect of our perception of beauty may have to do with the seduction of vital power, of raw, radiant life made manifest to the eyes.

This is why I began the chapter with an epigraph from Ruskin's *Queen of the Air*. The passage cited concludes a longer rhapsody on the spirit of plants:

> [T]he power that catches out of chaos charcoal, water, lime or what not and fastens down into a given form, is properly called "spirit"; and we shall not diminish but strengthen our conception of this creative energy by recognizing its presence in lower states of matter than our own; such recognition being enforced upon us by delight we instinctively receive from all the forms of matter which manifest it; and yet more, by the glorifying of those forms, in the parts of them that are most animated, with the colors that are pleasantest to our senses. The most familiar instance of this is the best, and also the most wonderful: the blossoming of plants.
>
> The spirit in the plant — that is to say its power of gathering dead matter out of the wreck round it, and shaping it into its own chosen shape — is of course strongest at the moment of its flowering, for it then not only gathers, but forms, with the greatest energy.[95]

Ruskin's accent on shapes and creative formation recalls some of the habits of seeing that we encountered before in Greek anatomy. But in his perception of blossoming hues as the purest expression of vital power, in his association of life, rapture, and flushed color, Ruskin also imparts some insight into the nature and depth of response that *se* elicited in China.

Greek physicians, too, acknowledged parallels between animals (including human animals) and plants. While voluntary motion separated the zoological from the botanical realm, both animals and plants nourished themselves and grew. This is why growth and nutrition were deemed functions of the vegetative soul.[96] The drying out of the body in old age, says Galen, is like the withering of plants.[97] In China, however, botanical analogy

189

didn't just illuminate select lower aspects of the human economy. It defined as well the innermost core of the heart.

To defend the doctrine that later became the cornerstone of Confucian orthodoxy — the essential goodness of human nature — Mencius turned to the lessons of plants. All humans, he affirmed, are born good. But the four qualities that express this goodness — benevolence, rightness, rites, and wisdom — are like four incipient shoots (*si duan*). To nurture them, to insure their full development, one must constantly attend to them. Yet one cannot *force* them to grow. The cultivation of the self, like the cultivation of plants, differs from the exertion involved in, say, moving a rock. It isn't a matter of just deciding, and then pushing or pulling. It isn't a matter of muscular resolve. Witness the folly of the man from Song:

> There was a man from Song who pulled at his rice plants because he was worried about their failure to grow. Having done so, he went on his way home, not realizing what he had done. "I am worn out today," said he to his family. "I have been helping the rice plants to grow." His son rushed out to take a look and there the plants were, all shrivelled up.[98]

The last chapter uncovered ties between the Greek vision of the body and two forms of self-assertion: the articulation of intentions and the exercise of muscular will. Chinese self-definition appealed to neither. Far more influential in China was the metaphor of the growth and flourishing of plants. Here is the deeper sense in which the scrutiny of *se* matched the contemplation of blooming flowers. Humans resembled plants not just in "vegetative" processes, such as growth and nutrition, but in their moral development, in the way they grew and revealed themselves as persons.

190

Because the flowering visage (*huase*) is the bloom of the body's essences, declares the *Suwen*, "In someone of virtue, the *qi* appears calm in the eye, and one knows by the face the conquest of sorrow."[99] The face is the flowering of feeling, says the *Guoyu*; and conversely, "Flower," according to a common gloss, "is *se*" (*hua se ye*). "Benevolence, rightness, the rites, and wisdom," Mencius observes, "are rooted (*gen*) in the heart and give rise to an expression (*se*) that appears pure and luminous in the face (*mao*)."[100] *Se* expressed the person much as blossoms express the plant.

In his book on the intellectual and social background of Chinese science, Derk Bodde observes that, "[S]ince very early times the Chinese were apparently much more interested in crops and plants than in animals." He then cites Ho Ping-ti's observation that: "Throughout China's long historic periods the agricultural system ... has always been lopsided in favor of grain production, with animal husbandry playing a subsidiary role.... The Chinese had yet another peculiar trait, namely, the unusually late beginning and persistent underutilization of draft animals for cultivation."[101]

These remarks tantalize with vague hints of how socioeconomic factors may have shaped the history of medical seeing. Greek anatomy, we know, revolved around animals: not only were they the victims of most dissections, but the very idea of dissection owed much to curiosity about their organizing logic. A major inspiration for inquiry into musculature, moreover, was the desire to illuminate the secrets of animation, to clarify the wonderful capacity for self-movement which made animals, including human animals, distinct from plants. Ancient Greek botany bred no comparable will to anatomize.

As an object, the body is unlike any other. It is the unique, intimately felt site of personal identity. Queries like, How did Chinese (or Greek) doctors imagine the structure of the body? —

191

or, How did they think the body worked? — thus can never fully solve, by themselves, the puzzling contrast between envisioning muscularity and gazing at *se*. For the puzzle is only partially about contrasting ideas of anatomy and physiology. It also involves diverging perceptions of persons, disparities in how people see and experience their own being. Articulate musculature, on the one hand, on the other, flourishing hues. Alternate visions of the body reflect alternate readings of the vital self.

And yet about the substance of vitality, Greek and Chinese doctors agreed. Both traced life's power to blood and breath. Which leads us to wonder: How did this shared sense of life's rootedness in blood and breath mesh with the diverging views of vitality manifest in muscles and in *se*? Our inquiries into the pulse and the *mo* have whispered to us from the start that knowing the body was inseparable from a feel for blood and breath.

PART THREE

Styles of Being

CHAPTER FIVE

Blood and Life

Therapeutic bleeding has virtually vanished today. The sick are no longer covered with leeches or bled to unconsciousness. Did such cures once actually heal and revitalize? Current opinion accuses them instead of weakening, even killing. The very idea of nurturing life by draining blood has come to seem hopelessly barbaric, absurd.

Yet for a great part of Western history most doctors felt otherwise. Galen let blood for such sundry ailments as gout and arthritis, dizziness and blackouts, epilepsy, melancholy, peripneumonia, pleurisy, liver disease, opthalmia, and even hemorrhages — to list merely a few. He declared phlebotomy "an essential remedy," called for "in any severe disease,"[1] and he supposed this faith to be entirely traditional. The great physicians before him, he maintained, had also esteemed bleeding as a cure equal "to the most effective of all."[2]

Medieval healers were no less enthusiastic, regularly bleeding the healthy as well the sick, to insure optimal vigor.[3] Embraced as "the great beginning of health," bloodletting promised a limitless horizon of virtues: "It makes the mind sincere, it aids the memory, it purges the brain, it reforms the bladder, it warms the marrow, it opens the hearing, it checks tears, it removes nausea, it

195

benefits the stomach, it invites digestion, it evokes the voice, it builds up the sense, it moves the bowels, it enriches sleep, it removes anxiety. . . ."[4] "A bleeding in the spring is physic for a king," summarized an old English adage.[5]

Nor did faith decline in the seventeenth century, with the discovery of blood's circulation. William Harvey himself prized bleeding as the "foremost among all the general remedial means."[6] And in the eighteenth century, Lorenz Heister's popular textbook of surgery continued to favor phlebotomy among procedures performed on the whole body. "We begin with the operation of phlebotomy," Heister explained, "because it is of all [operations] the most general, performed in most parts of the body, and by much the most frequent in use at the present day."[7] Even in 1839, Marshall Hall, whose critique of indiscriminate phlebotomy allegedly helped spur bloodletting's eventual decline, conceded nonetheless that of the therapies available to the physician in his time, it "ranked preeminently as the first."[8]

Some thirty years later, the naturalist Charles Waterton still relied on phlebotomy as the cornerstone of prophylaxis. Since the age of twenty-four, he relates, he had been bled no less than a hundred and ten times and had bled himself in eighty of those instances. This was how he had kept himself "in as perfect health as a man can be" while trekking through distant jungles.[9]

In this long and remarkable tradition, we glimpse a fundamental yet little-noticed difference between the histories of Western and Chinese medicine. From antiquity through the mid-nineteenth century, the letting of blood flourished as one of the most common and trusted means of caring for the body — in the West.[10] But not in China.

What does this contrast mean? Because of its centrality in the history of Western therapeutics, and because of Hippocrates' reputation as the source of medical wisdom, scholars have sometimes traced the zeal for bleeding back to the physician of Cos. No less an authority than Emile Littré opined that, "When we inquire which remedies among the many that were used, are most frequently mentioned as having been applied, we find that bloodletting and the evacuants...play the principal role in the therapy of the Hippocratic physicians, and hence of Hippocrates himself."[11]

However, with respect to bloodletting at least, the evidence suggests otherwise. The approximately seventy references to letting blood in the Hippocratic corpus earn it only a small place on the map of Hippocratic therapeutics. No treatises or even extended passages develop an explicit theory of phlebotomy. As Peter Brain concluded, the idea that Hippocratic physicians touted bloodletting as the most effective of remedies is a myth.[12] Bleeding became a prime pillar of Western medicine only later, after Hippocrates.

Galen devoted no less than three lengthy works to venesection (*On Venesection*, *On Venesection Against Erasistratus*, and *On Venesection Against the Erasistrateans*), elaborating in these and other writings a theory of the body and its afflictions which made bleeding both the preferred treatment for a wide range of disorders, and the chief tool of prophylaxis. Attitudes had changed.

So there is a history to bloodletting. Galen speaks of the great trust placed in bleeding by his predecessors, including Hippocrates, but his own fervor colors his view of history. Celsus' remarks on the situation in his time (circa 30 C.E.) are at least suggestive. "It is not new to let blood by cutting a vein," he observes, "but that there is hardly any disease in which blood is not let, is new."[13]

Long before the development of acupuncture needles — a development which Yamada Keiji dates to the Western Han — Chinese healers punctured abscesses and let blood with bladed-stone

197

or bronze scalpels called *bianshi*.[14] So bloodletting wasn't unknown in ancient China. On the contrary. References to it still abound in the *Neijing*, and one modern scholar has even described bleeding as the *main* therapy promoted in the work.[15]

By the late Han dynasty, however, recourse to the remedy had apparently declined. The *Nanjing*, the canonical classic written to elucidate crucial topics from the *Neijing*, doesn't mention it at all, and references to the cure appear only sporadically in later works. D.C. Epler discerns, more subtly, a shift in attitudes already within the *Neijing* itself. Focusing specifically on the *Suwen*, he has reconstructed an evolution whereby the bloodletting promoted in the older sections of this compilation disappears in the newer treatises.[16]

Ancient Chinese therapeutics thus evolved in almost the exact opposite direction from the Greek. Once a major cure, bleeding lost its popularity after the *Neijing*. Not that it died out altogether: among the exotica collected in the *Taiping guangji* (978), for instance, is the record of how a doctor cured the Tang emperor Gaozong of a severe headache and blurred vision by letting blood from the top of his head;[17] and Gao Wu's compendium of acupuncture, the *Zhenjiu juying* (1519), notes that the renowned physician Li Gao sometimes let blood from acupuncture sites (though he did this, significantly, with an explicit consciousness of returning to the classical example of the *Neijing*).[18] For a few afflictions, particularly those marked by skin eruptions, such as leprosy and *sha* disorders, bloodletting even counted among standard treatments.[19] Still, viewed against the whole of postclassical medical therapeutics, the references to bloodletting figure as little more than rare and scattered exceptions.

In the history of bloodletting, just as in the history of palpation, comparison across traditions proves inseparable from the study of change within each tradition.[20] There was a time when

Greek and Chinese healers alike let blood, and did so, we shall see, in intriguingly similar ways. But then their attitudes toward bloodletting traced sharply diverging trajectories.

Blood and Life

Haunting concerns about blood appear early in both Greek and Chinese writings. But then again, our own discomfort with blood-letting derives partly from an intuition that is doubtless prehistoric, namely, that blood is essential to life. Lose enough of it, and we die. We imagine this confirmed daily in the slaughter of animals, and in the carnage of war. The association between the loss of blood from wounds and the ebbing of life presumably underlies the kinship between Homer's word for gore, *brótos*, and his term for mortal, *brotós*. The gods, immortal, *ambrotoi*, are not made of the same stuff. The Furies track down Orestes by the smell of his blood, and seek to suck it out of him as payment for the life that he has taken. "The life of every creature," Leviticus teaches, "is the blood of it."[21]

Yet we would expect this equation of life and blood to lead away from, rather than toward, the practice of bloodletting. And in fact, most phlebotomists avoided bleeding fragile patients — young children and the elderly, for instance — while some physicians, like van Helmont in the Renaissance, rejected bloodletting altogether, arguing precisely that in draining blood the healer drained the patient's soul.[22] That bloodletting thrived despite the claims of blood as life bespeaks the pull of other considerations. Two merit special note.

One is the observation that life isn't sustained by blood alone, that breath is also vital. The departure of breath is expiration, death. In both classical Greek and Chinese medicine, life-sustaining vessels distributed breath — *qi* and *pneuma* — as well as blood.

A second factor was the belief that blood and breath deter-

199

mined not just *whether* one lived, but *how*. Their power was necessary for even the most elementary activities. Thus it is blood received in the liver, the *Neijing* asserts, that allows one to see, blood in the foot that enables one to walk, blood in the palm that makes grasping possible, and blood in the fingers that gives touch.[23] More generally, qualities of blood and breath governed qualities of life. Recall Confucius's account of the "three things that the superior man guards against": "When he is young and the blood and breath are not yet settled, he guards against lust. When he matures, and the blood and breath are in full vigor, he guards against combativeness. When he is old, and the blood and breath have declined, he guards against covetousness."[24]

Changes in blood and breath alter impulses and inclinations. From blood and breath spring desire, and aggression, and greed. Anger and fear too, according to Chinese doctors: the former results from a suffusion of blood, the latter from its lack.[25] Greek writers evinced similar intuitions. The boiling of blood around the heart gave rise to the "spirit," or *thumos*, in Homer's heroes; Empedocles held that "The blood around men's hearts is their thought."[26]

Blood also affects susceptibility to sickness. According to one Hippocratic treatise, adults suffer little from the blockage of blood vessels by phlegm because their blood vessels "are capacious and full of hot blood; as a result, the phlegm cannot gain the upper hand and chill and freeze the blood." Likewise, the very old rarely die from phlegm blockage, but for the opposite reason: their "vessels are empty and the blood small in quantity and of thin and watery consistency."[27] Close ties between blood and sickness explain as well why, in Galen's view, women menstruating normally don't suffer severe illnesses, whereas all kinds of disorders arise from suppressed menses.[28] Disruptions in blood and breath, the *Neijing* concludes, evolve into the hundred diseases.[29]

While the identification of blood with vitality sometimes militated against bloodletting, the association of qualities of blood and qualities of life made blood a compelling target of cures. Too much blood, too little blood, blood that is too hot or too cold, blood that races through vessels or is trapped and stagnant, imbalances in the distribution of blood, bad blood — all these affect what a person can do, how a person feels, who a person is.[30] Some of these conditions were treated by letting blood.

Topological Bleeding

The first question that confronts the would-be phlebotomist, Galen suggests, is this: "[W]hether it makes no difference which vein is opened, as some think, or whether there are special veins for each of the affected parts. ..."[31] Galen presents the problem as one on which "extensive research has been undertaken."[32] Bloodletting guided by the latter view — that one bleeds particular veins to treat particular parts of the body — is what I shall call topological bleeding.

Galen asserts that "Hippocrates and the most celebrated physicians" promoted topological bleeding,[33] and the Hippocratic corpus bears him out. References to bloodletting regularly prescribe specific sites to bleed. "Dysuria is cured by bleeding, and the incision should be in the inner vein."[34] To relieve afflictions of the liver, one must let blood from the right elbow; for afflictions of the spleen, from the left elbow;[35] for pains in the back, from veins on the outside of the ankles; for testicular pains, from the inside of the ankles.[36] Different ailments required bleeding different sites. *Where* one drew blood was critical.

Why? The word *phleps* (plural: *phlebes*) is often translated as "vein." But *phlebes* were not veins in the modern sense, i.e., veins as opposed to arteries. Veins and arteries were first distinguished by Hellenistic dissectors, well after Hippocrates. Nor did *phlebes*

refer simply to arteries and veins together — to a vague, undifferentiated intuition of blood vessels, merely innocent of anatomy's fine discriminations. As described in Hippocratic treatises such as the *Sacred Disease*, *Nature of the Human Being*, *Nature of Bones*, and *Places in the Human Being*, and in Aristotle's *History of Animals*, the paths of the *phlebes* depart, often wildly, from the paths of the arteries and veins that we know today.[37] *Phlebes* were not just anatomically indiscriminate; they were anatomically false. If we limit the truth of the body to the truths of dissection, the *phlebes* appear like fantasies.[38]

Yet we know — for the ancient accounts tell us explicitly, and casually, as if they were nothing remarkable — what kinds of experiences once supported belief in these veins: the topology of the *phlebes* went hand-in-hand with the topology of bloodletting. Their strange paths mirrored a grasp of bodily connectedness rooted not in the scrutiny of the dead, but in the care of the living.

One had to bleed the right elbow for liver pain, and the left for spleen problems, because the vein in the right elbow ran to the liver, whereas that in the left elbow led directly to the spleen. This was the logic of site-specificity: to treat an affliction in a particular part of the body, one bled the vein that served that part. Choosing the proper vein was especially critical since no theory of vasculature in ancient Greece posited a continuous circulation.[39] The *phlebes* irrigated the body as largely independent channels, with few interconnections. Letting blood from one *phleps* might thus be useless, even harmful, in treating parts or organs served by another.

Hippocratic physicians could thus justify topological bleeding by appealing to the structure of the veins. Of course, the original order of discovery may have actually been the reverse. We could suppose that healers first observed the effects of bleeding from certain sites on other, remote parts of the body, and from these

observations elaborated a net of linking channels. Most likely, theories of veins and practices of bleeding evolved together, with inferences running both ways. In any case, Hippocratic *phlebes* were not crude anticipations of the arteries and veins of later anatomy. Rather, they expressed an alternative approach to the body, one which envisioned somatic structure through the topology of pain and its relief.

Current discourse on pain focuses on the brain and nerves. We learn that in those parts where nerves are few, or absent, or dead, we feel little or no hurt. Our cures block neural pathways, or more colloquially, "deaden" the nerves. We hardly think of blood in connection with our aches and agonies, or we do so only in terms of wounds. But in Hippocrates, hemorrhaging was associated as often with *curing* pain as with causing it, and pain relief was the prime motive for the letting of blood.

In ancient China, too, bleeding often aimed to quell pain. Harmful breaths lodged in the Lesser Yin *mo* running up from the foot, explains the *Suwen*, cause heart pain, violent swellings, fullness of the chest, flanks, and limbs. The cure? Bleeding from near the source of the *mo*, in front of the inner ankle.[40] Back pain offers a particularly telling case. If the pain stretches all along the back from the nape of the neck to the buttocks, then one should bleed from the *xizhong* site of the Greater Yang *mo* — what we now call the popliteal vein, at the back of the knee. On the other hand, back pain in which the patient is unable to roll over should be treated by bleeding from the *wailian* site of the Lesser Yang *mo*. Other types of back pain required bleeding from yet other sites, for each *mo* traversed a different region of the back.[41]

Let blood from one part of a vessel to solve suffering in another part. Let blood from the leg or arm to relieve pain in the head, say, or the liver. We find the same principle also in Hippocrates. Sometimes, Chinese and Greek treatments even coincide: doctors in both traditions thus bled the back of the knee for back pain. A number of Hippocratic cures, moreover, such as bleeding the inner ankle for testicular pain, have close analogues in acupuncture. Though the match between the paths of the *phlebes* and the *mo* is nowhere exact, the two arguably share more with each other than with the arteries and veins defined by dissection. Early on, Greek and Chinese physicians articulated the bonds between blood and pain through conduits that are tantalizingly alike.

Which suggests two arresting possibilities.

One is that acupuncture may have evolved out of bloodletting.[42] Probably not *just* from bloodletting, of course: the earliest extant medical accounts of the *mo*, remember, refer neither to bleeding or needling, but only to moxibustion. Still, as we noted in chapter 1, the idea of the *mo* was originally intertwined with the blood vessels visible at the body surface, and it was from these *mo* that the *jingluo* pathways of acupuncture developed. Many crucial needling points lie on surface veins and arteries, and we sometimes find the same sites deployed in both acupuncture and in bloodletting to treat a given hurt.

The second possibility is that of a genetic kinship between developments in ancient Greece and China. The movement of peoples and goods between the eastern and western reaches of Eurasia is prehistoric, and it isn't hard to conceive of a cure such as drawing blood from the knee for back pain migrating across the continent. We know in particular that the Scythians and other nomadic peoples ranged widely across Eurasia, and that they had fairly extensive contact with both Greek and Chinese cultures. We know, too, from *Airs, Waters, Places,* that the Scythians, like the Greeks and Chinese, cauterized and let blood. Most significantly, we know that Scythian bloodletting presupposed ties between remote parts of the body — ties that evince surprising parallels to those posited by the early Greeks and Chinese. To treat varicose veins and lameness, the nomads let blood not locally, from the legs, as one might expect, but from "the vein behind each ear."[43]

To be sure, the kinship between Greek and Chinese practices could be explained in a quite different way. We could suppose that healers in the two traditions drew blood from similar sites for similar afflictions because doing so actually produced relief. The commonality in treatment might be rooted, that is, in the commonality of human physiology.

Modern historians of medicine have generally been skeptical of bloodletting's efficacy. While aggressive condemnation is now fairly rare, attempts to justify the cure physiologically are even rarer.[44] Bloodletting's past popularity has usually been attributed, instead, to cultural or psychological factors, such as the doctrinal authority and coherence of Galenic humoralism, the psychosomatic power of the patient's faith, and the logic of the traditional patient-healer relationship.[45] Peter Murray Jones's view of medieval practice reflects the general trend: "Most bloodletting done on a regular basis was quite safe and probably provided psychological reassurance *if nothing else*, but some of the bloodletting undertaken in the treatment of illnesses very likely did much more harm than good, and must have caused unnecessary deaths in extreme cases" (italics added). [46]

Whether such skepticism is justified I cannot say. Certainly no one would deny the impact of cultural and psychological expectations on therapies of any kind. Nevertheless, the parallels between topological bleeding and acupuncture should give us pause.

By a curious irony, many in the West today readily concede the possibility of an empirical basis for the exotic technique of acupuncture, while they dismiss offhand the phlebotomy practiced assiduously in Europe for over two millennia. Yet as we've just seen, acupuncture and topological bleeding were actually kindred techniques, positing similar, sometimes identical connections between sites of treatment and distant ailing parts. To the extent that we willingly entertain the possibility of some physiological rationale for acupuncture, we may also need to rethink bloodletting.

In any event, accounting for *why* Chinese and Hippocratic bloodletting display similarities is less critical for our inquiry than just recognizing *that* they do. For the backdrop of this early congruence between Greek and Chinese therapies permits us to define more crisply the nature and magnitude of the subsequent changes. Once upon a time, Greek and Chinese physicians alike let blood topologically. By the end of the ancient period, this tantalizing resemblance would give way to therapies so different that few would suspect the kinship between them.

The Evolution of Greek Phlebotomy

Two notable changes occurred in Greek phlebotomy between the times of Hippocrates and Galen. One was the emergence of doubts about topological bleeding; the other was the transformation of phlebotomy into a cornerstone of therapy.

The issue raised by Galen's first question of phlebotomy — whether it matters from which vein one lets blood — reflects a skepticism about topological bleeding in late antiquity which we don't find in Hippocratic texts. The majority of Hippocratic references to phlebotomy specify the particular site that should be bled. Even in the case of spontaneous nosebleeds, doctors note carefully whether blood flows from the left nostril or the right nostril, or both. For both diagnosis and therapy, the divide between right and left was critical. No Hippocratic doctor would say that the choice of veins didn't matter.

Yet this was just the thesis, Galen tells us, advanced by some of his contemporaries.[47] While there were still those, like Galen himself, who rejected this view,[48] sufficient uncertainty had arisen about old practices to inspire "extensive research" and to make the relevance of vein selection the most pressing problem of phlebotomy.

Not that topological bleeding suffered sudden, definitive decline. It had, after all, no less eminent an advocate than Galen, and at least some attention to sites persisted throughout the entire history of bloodletting.[49] Nonetheless, the bleeding practices of someone like Aretaeus (81–138) already displays a distinct skepticism about traditional site selection.[50]

What lay behind this shift? Again, the rise of dissection likely played a role. Anatomical inspection undercut topological bleeding by exposing discrepancies between the paths posited for the Hippocratic *phlebes* and the anatomy of arteries and veins.[51] More fundamentally, it brought to the fore a new conception of connectedness, a conception based not on inferences drawn from physiological response, but on the continuities seen in the corpse. Doctors could still argue that for evacuating blood from a given organ some veins were more efficient than others — by virtue of their structural proximity; and it was on just these grounds that apologists like Galen defended topological bleeding all while rejecting previous theories of the *phlebes*.[52] But this argument wasn't always possible. And so from late antiquity onward an uneasy tension persisted throughout the history of Western medicine between the claims of anatomy and the bleeding practices sanctioned by tradition.[53]

A second major development that made site selection seem less urgent was the increasing tendency, after Hippocrates, to equate phlebotomy with the release of excess blood. In defending topological bleeding, Galen suggests that "the proper study of physicians" must include knowing "when one should cut the vein in the forehead, and when those at the corners of the eyes, or under the tongue, the one known as the shoulder vein, or the one through the axilla, or the veins in the hams or alongside the ankle."[54]

He insists on this, however, not so much against critics who actively denied the meaningfulness of site differentiation, but against those who neglected sites because they believed "that one should simply let blood from patients who are at risk of a *plethos*" — an idea which Galen characterizes as "not worthy of Hippocrates' art."[55] This brings me to one of my main theses: the transformation of bloodletting from a relatively minor remedy into an indispensable pillar of Greek therapeutics turned, I suggest, on the fear of plethora. Underlying the devotion to phlebotomy was the dread of excess blood.

Elaborating this hypothesis requires some care. Many of the core intuitions about plethora can be glimpsed already in Hippocrates.[56] My thesis is thus less about the birth of new ideas than about the crystallization of an altered consciousness. While Hippocrates hardly spoke of plethora, Galen invoked the term at every turn. This change in discourse signaled a new awareness of the body and its role in sickness, a shift in etiological focus. It is this shift that I want ultimately to elucidate. But let me start with the core ideas.

Hippocratic physicians often assert that menstruation and other forms of hemorrhage, such as hemorrhoids and bleeding from the nose (*epistaxis*), have curative and prophylactic value. *Epidemics* 1 reports, for instance, that during a certain epidemic,

> Though many women fell ill, they were fewer than the men and less frequently died.... Some bled from the nose. Sometimes both epis-

taxis and menstruation appeared together.... I know of no woman who died if any of these symptoms showed themselves properly.[57]

And again,

the most likely patients to survive were those who had a proper and copious bleeding from the nose. In fact, I do not know of a single case in this constitution that proved fatal when a proper bleeding occurred.[58]

Epidemics 6 adds that those with hemorrhoids are free of pleurisy and peripneumonia and a series of other afflictions.[59] *Coan Prognosis* suggests that the passing of blood with stools helps relieve cardiac, hepatic, and periumbilical pains.[60]

Conversely, the absence or suppression of such desirable hemorrhages can cause vicious harm. *Coan Prognosis* warns that the retention of blood in amenorrhea can induce epilepsy.[61] *Epidemics* 4 tells of a patient who ignored his doctor's advice not to have his hemorrhoids treated, and consequently raved mad.[62] And the treatise *On Wounds* recommends drawing blood quickly from contusions and open wounds, for blood accumulating around an injury can become heated and putrefy and thus give rise to inflammations, pus, and ulcers.[63]

As for the origin of blood, *Diseases* 4 traces it directly to food. This explains why, directly after a meal, the jugular veins swell and the face reddens.[64] This influx of material must eventually be eliminated through excretions or bleeding — Greek authors habitually treat diarrhea and hemorrhage, purgation, fasting, and venesection as having comparable effects — otherwise disease ensues. Normally, the body conquers food and food makes it grow; but sometimes food conquers the body, producing a wide array of sicknesses.[65]

All these Hippocratic observations — the dangers of excess blood, the therapeutic usefulness of natural and artificial hemorrhages, the origins of blood in food, and the tendency of blood to putrefy and cause inflammation — find their way into Galen's concept of plethora. Yet the review I've just given is misleading. In Hippocrates the ideas appear only as scattered remarks; Galen gives them ample, systematic development. This might seem a consequence of the fact that bloodletting was central to Galenic therapy and only peripheral to Hippocratic healing. But I believe that the arrow of causation points mainly in the opposite direction: it was the new, urgent stress on some traditional ideas that made bloodletting seem vital to the prevention and cure of disease.

Even in Galen's time not all bloodletting aimed to relieve plethora. Galen himself explicitly rejects this view of the remedy. "Menodotus is wrong," he argues, "in saying that phlebotomy should be approved only in the syndrome known as the plethoric."

> The indications for phlebotomy do not primarily include *plethos*, but the suspicion that disease is developing. If it appears that it will be severe, we shall invariably phlebotomize, even if none of the signs of *plethos* is present....
>
> [T]he first and most important indications for phlebotomy are... the severity of the disease and the strength of the patient, and it is necessary to say that this, and not the plethoric syndrome, is the principal combination of circumstances for which phlebotomy has been approved.[66]

Often, then, one must let blood even in the absence of *plethos*. Galen is insistent about this.[67] Yet some, like Menodotus, clearly

did equate bloodletting with relieving plethora, and Galen's repeated rejection of this equation suggests that this was a widespread, perhaps even standard perception.

Understood properly, moreover, Galen's critique actually reinforces, rather than severs, the link between phlebotomy and
plethora. For what he decries is a myopic preoccupation with the
patient's immediate condition, with whether plethora exists at
the moment. In his view, phlebotomy serves not only to relieve
an existing excess of blood, but also, and more effectively, to *prevent* such excess from forming. The wise physician, ever mindful
of plethora's menace, lets blood prophylactically, before an excess
can accumulate.[68] Immediate bleeding is thus sometimes called
for even in the absence of a general plethos, such as when someone suffers a blow or pain — "for pain attracts blood."[69]

Concern about excess blood wasn't confined to advocates of
phlebotomy. Erasistratus, Galen relates, also urged "people to
keep the closest watch on their health, by knowing in advance
how to recognize and to guard against the condition of plethora."
Doctors strove to head off plethora "when it is approaching, before the illness has begun."[70] Erasistratus apparently shunned
bloodletting, however, and instead championed fasting.[71] Hence
the logic of starving a fever: "[When] illnesses are beginning and
the onset of inflammatory conditions, all sloppy foods should be
withdrawn together with solids, for the inflammations that give
rise to fevers arise for the most part as a result of plethora. If
nourishment is given at such times and digestion and distribution
perform their functions, the vessels are filled with nutriment and
more powerful inflammations will ensue."[72]

So there was some disagreement about the best remedy for
plethora. While acknowledging the general usefulness of fasting,
Galen objected that in many cases bleeding was the more efficient, even the only effective cure.[73] But both he and Erasistratus

concurred about the urgency of treatment, and for us this is the crucial point. The relative merits of fasting versus bleeding concern us less than the fact that these two practices — the former still assiduously practiced today, though its uses and ostensible rationale have changed, and the latter now largely condemned and forgotten — were traditionally viewed as very nearly equivalent. Fasting reduced the intake of food, the latter eliminated its residues.[74] Though approaching the problem from opposite ends, both mirrored the obsession with excess blood.

Plethora gripped the Greek imagination with an intensity that the bare logic of intake and consumption cannot explain. Physicians sometimes exsanguinated their patients until they fainted and passed feces, so terrible was the perceived danger. Plethora was excess, and thus pathological by definition. But contrary to what we would expect (were balance per se the supreme concern), depletion, plethora's opposite, provoked no comparable anxious vigilance. The compulsion to bleed was inseparable from the fear of excess blood. Galen is explicit: the best preparation for studying his *Treatment by Venesection*, he advises, is to read his essay on plethora.[75]

Stagnant hot plethoric excess putrefied and inflamed, made even good blood bilious, generated fevers.[76] One had to bleed quickly, before inflammation (*phlegmonē*) set in. Forestalling inflammation was key.[77]

Inflammation arose, Galen thought, from the flux of blood. A wound or fracture could induce the flux, but it might also result from the diversion of a general plethora into some part "most apt to receive" the excess blood. The humoral mix determined the character of the resultant inflammation: blood in which yellow bile predominated produced *herpēs*; very hot bile, *erysipelas*; hot thick blood, *anthrax*; phlegm, *oidēma*. A mixture of black bile and

212

blood caused an inflammation known as *scirrhus*, one form of which could become cancer. A flux of pure black bile produced cancers (*karkina*).[78] If the Greeks worried far more about inflammation than we do, it was in part because the concept had greater range.

Galen's concept of inflammation encompassed cancerous lesions, benign tumors, and inflammatory growths. Consequently, his *Preternatural Tumors* (*Peri tōn para physin onkōn*) is really more about what we would consider inflammations than about true tumors (*onkoi*) in the modern sense.[79] Before François Bichat's tissue theory and Johannes Mueller's application of cell theory to pathology, neoplasms, benign tumors, and inflammatory growths were all traced to concentrations of corrupt blood.

Looking at "inflammations" in this way, we begin to appreciate the urgency with which ancient physicians sought to prevent them. Greek physicians recognized that once established, many cancers were fatal; salvation lay in early intervention or, better, prophylaxis. Timely bleeding saved lives. But it would be anachronistic to reduce the ancient obsession with plethora to contemporary fears of cancer. Cancer didn't loom as large in antiquity as it does now, because most people succumbed sooner to other sicknesses, before they reached the ages when cancer claims its most victims.

Ultimately, the gnawing anxieties about plethora were rooted not so much in the gravity of particular diseases, but in the intuition that plethora was responsible for virtually *all* disease.

In culling evidence for Hippocratic views on bleeding I cited several passages from *Epidemics* 1. But in fact remarks on the problem of blood retention and the benefits of blood release form only a minor part of the treatise's observations about causes and cures. The work lavishes more attention on factors that we tend presently to forget — factors such as seasonal weather and wind.

Galen asserts by contrast that, "Whatever sickens the body from internal evil has a twofold explanation, either plethora or dyspepsia."[80] The latter results from eating improper foods or an unbalanced diet; the former from taking in more nutriment than is either consumed by the body in its activities or evacuated in wastes. Taken by themselves, Galen's remarks might seem merely to complement Hippocratic environmentalism — to address the internal causes of disease, while treatises like *Epidemics 1* and *Airs, Waters, Places* described the external circumstances. But in Galenic analysis, the body's inner state was absolutely fundamental: the presence or absence of internal evil largely determined the harm caused by external elements.

Foreshadowing later ideas of germs, for example, Galen refers to "pestilential seeds" (*loimou spermata*) of disease. He is interested, however, less in the nature of the seeds per se than in the question of why some people succumb to pestilence while others don't. His conclusion is unequivocal. "We must always remember ... this principle: that none of the causes [of disease] can operate without a predisposition in the patient." And again, "The greatest part of the generation of disease lies in the preparation of the body." Inhaling pathogens doesn't, in itself, cause sickness. Pestilential seeds take root and grow only in a body predisposed to corruption, a body already made full by overeating, indolence, and sexual indulgence. A plethoric body.[81]

While the theory of the seeds of disease commanded only a minor place in Galen's pathology (he mentions it in only a few passages),[82] the same belief in the primacy of inner states also undergirded his analysis of the most basic form of external affliction, namely, wounds. Sometimes, he observes, a prick from a very fine needle can induce a huge inflammation. The manifest disparity here between the apparent cause and the effect proves that the chief culprit is actually not the needle but the body into which it enters. If a tiny wound swells massively with pus, it must be because of a preexisting plethora of unevacuated residues.[83] In bodies without excess, even large gashes heal quickly, without inflammation and festering.[84] Even in the paradigmatic case of external causation, then, even when a patient suffers cuts or blows, the extent of damage hinges ultimately on the body's internal complexion—hinges, that is, on plethora or its absence.

How does one recognize plethora? We could have predicted some of the indications: a ruddy complexion, distended veins, a large pulse, and a history of physical inactivity, excessive eating and drinking, suppressed evacuations. What is remarkable about Galen's diagnosis of plethora, however, is his stress on the patient's own feelings. The symptoms on which he puts the most weight are heaviness in the whole body, sluggishness, tension in the limbs, pain, and lassitude.[85] One recognizes plethora, in other words, not just through objective signs such as the pulse, but also and above all in a person's subjective experience of the body.

Heaviness, inertia, tension, pain. These are familiar sensations. At different times, to varying degrees, we all experience them. And this suggests how plethora could once have seemed so widespread, and the need for bloodletting so routine. Scanning the people around us we may spot a few red-faced individuals whom we might judge plethoric; but mostly, it's hard for us to imagine excess blood as anything but a rare oddity. This is part of what makes past enthusiasm for bloodletting seem so strange. On the other hand, once we turn from the abstract notion of excess blood to the symptoms that supposedly announce it, the condition assumes a more intimate cast. Though we may never have thought ourselves plethoric, we know what it is to feel heavy and sluggish, or to suffer from tense, aching muscles.

Plethora was thus a disease not only in the detached, clinical sense of humoral imbalance, but also the dis-ease of subjective discomfort, the nagging claim of the body on consciousness. Galen speaks frequently of the heaviness (*barutēs*) of the plethoric body, by which he refers not to its absolute weight, but to the sensation of sluggishness in a body that responds but slowly and grudgingly to the will. His descriptions curiously echo character-izations of the body that we find in Plato, a thinker he greatly admired.

The soul that follows God and obtains sight of the truth, Socrates declares, is freed from all harm; but the soul that cannot follow and fails to see is "filled with forgetfulness and evil, and grows heavy, and when it has grown heavy ... falls to the earth."[86] Evil's heavy weight, though, is none other than the burden of the body. Whereas the soul naturally aspires upward to the heavens and to the Good, the body is "burdensome, heavy, and earthly," and weighs it down.[87]

Especially suggestive here is the origin of blood in food. An old belief had it that the soul could occasionally escape its impris-onment in the darkness of the material body and regain its natural clairvoyance. In sleep, for instance; hence the prescience of dreams. Special diets, on the other hand, transformed the body itself, making it more transparent to psychic visions. Thus legends of the seer Epimenides speculated that he ate no earthly food, but nourished himself on the ethereal fare provided by nymphs.[88] After predicting the plague at Ephesus, Apollonius defended himself against charges of wizardry by tracing his foresight to an exceptionally light diet, which conferred a celestial clarity.[89] In his *Eclogae propheticae*, Clement of Alexandria forcefully advanced ties between fasting and spiritual possibility: "Fasting empties the soul of matter and makes it, with the body, clear and light for the reception of divine truth." Excessive food, "drags down the intel-

216

lectual part towards insensibility." Meals should thus always be plain and simple, to facilitate digestion and secure "lightness of the body."[90]

For Plato, the soul was light, luminous, and eternal, while the body was sluggish, dark, and corruptible; heaviness was intrinsic to the very condition of embodiment. For physicians, by contrast, the dull inertia of plethora was a temporary pathology—albeit a chronic danger. The coincidence between discourses thus wasn't exact. Still, clear echoes resonate between Galen's portrait of plethoric sluggishness and the plight of the Platonic soul imprisoned in flesh. The plethoric body was the body experienced when one was forced to become aware of it, when it ceased to be the easy instrument of will and desire and became a resistant onerous burden that weighed one down.

Emptiness in Chinese Medicine

Legends in ancient China told of sages who "avoided grains" (*bigu*), that is, shunned the coarse foods of ordinary mortals. Dwelling in misty mountains, they nourished themselves only on the fine pure breaths of high altitudes and enjoyed as a result extraordinary longevity and lightness of being. Reputedly, they floated around on clouds.

Here again, associations between light diet, light bodies, and sageliness—associations, moreover, which sometimes influenced actual regimen. Buried alongside the medical texts in the Mawangdui tombs, for instance, we find a treatise on "avoiding grains and feeding on vapors."[91] And the *Shiji* records that Zhang Liang, adviser to the first emperor of the Han dynasty, retired from politics specifically to devote himself to breathing exercises, the avoidance of grains, and the project of *qingshen*, lightening the body.[92]

Chinese medicine, however, developed no real equivalent to

Greek anxieties about plethora. Yes, food was the ultimate source of blood, and yes, too much food could swell the vessels and overflow in hemorrhages.[93] But the *Neijing* mentions nosebleeds and hemorrhoids only as disorders, never as salutary crises. Yes, doctors in China certainly condemned overeating, as they condemned excesses of any kind, and yes, they recognized complications arising from local congestions of blood. But they were never haunted by the prospect of a surfeit of blood burdening the body as a whole.

It is illuminating in this regard to consider a disorder about which they did voice concern and which offers some interesting resemblances to plethora. I mean *shi*. "Fullness" is a reasonable translation; expressions like *youyu* (surfeit), *man* (repletion), and *guo* (excess) often substituted as synonyms. As with plethora, the potential menace of *shi* was great: if not treated early, *shi* accumulations could grow into painful swellings, pustulent ulcers, ungainly excrescences, fatal tumors; as with plethora, the best treatment was prevention.[94] Furthermore, many of the common indications of *shi* — a full and hard *mo*, tension, pain, and fever — duplicated signs characteristic of plethora. A good part of the pathologies that Galen called plethoric his Chinese contemporaries would almost certainly have labeled *shi*.

But *shi* differed plainly from plethora in three respects. First, *shi* wasn't conceived primarily as a problem of blood. Second, fullness in China presupposed a necessary complement: nearly always, references to *shi* conjured up simultaneously the problem of *xu*, emptiness, and the two were typically yoked together as a compound, *xushi*, emptiness-and-fullness. Third, in this pairing of *xu* and *shi*, the former represented the more fundamental concern. If the excess of plethora was the guiding fear of the phlebotomist, Chinese reflections upon sickness began, contrarily, with depleted emptiness.

218

"Emptiness" and "fullness" in Chinese medicine each had two opposing meanings. In broad discussions of hygiene, emptiness named the deepest reality of being and the highest state of human spirituality. The Way (*dao*) is empty, Daoists rhapsodized, and so is the sage. Sagely emptiness was the emptiness of a mind detached from the senses, devoid of desire, lucid, limpid, serene.[95] Prized by some as itself the supreme end of self-cultivation, such emptiness was promoted by physicians as the final secret of vigor and longevity. It was only through a mind emptied of yearnings that one maintained a body full of vitality; to achieve fullness of life one had to abide in empty nothingness (*xuwu*).[96]

Unfortunately, most people failed to hold fast to this fullness. "The foolish never have enough [vitality]," the *Suwen* lamented, "the wise have an abundance."[97]

> The people of archaic times ... did not exhaust themselves capriciously. Thus it was possible for their bodies and their consciousness to be at one, so that they lived out their natural spans of life, passing away when their hundred years had been measured out.
>
> People of our times are not like that. Wine is their drink, caprice their norm. Drunken they enter the chamber of love, through lust using up their seminal essence, through desire dispersing their inborn vitality. They do not know how to maintain fullness (*buzhi chiman*). ... Lacking self-control in their activities, they are worn out at half a hundred.[98]

Most waste their lives. If fullness was health, then emptiness was sickness. This was the second and more common meaning of *xu* in medicine, the meaning that concerns us here: sickly depletion. Emptiness in this sense was pathological because it corresponded to diminished possibilities. The senses and limbs, which should remain alert and vigorous for a hundred years, already faltered at fifty. Bereft of vitality, the eyes and ears lost their acuity, the legs their spring, and hair turned prematurely gray. Worse, a depleted body was a vulnerable body, a body open to invasion. Pathological emptiness, *xu*, invited *shi*, pathological fullness.

> The Yellow Emperor asked, "What is meant by *xu* and *shi*?"
>
> Qi Bo replied, "When noxious breaths [from without] (*xieqi*) are ascendant, that is *shi*; when [a person's] essential breaths (*jingqi*) are depleted, that is *xu*.[99]

A mind devoid of desire, a body replete with vitality — these were emptiness and fullness as positive ideals of regimen. Most often, though, doctors spoke of emptiness and fullness as pathologies, of emptiness, that is, as depleted vitality, and of fullness as the state of a body filled by invasive evils.

What locked *xu* and *shi* together as pathologies, it is worth emphasizing, thus wasn't the symmetrical either-or logic of balance — the fear of exceeding or falling short of some abstract mean. No, the two were united rather by a hierarchy of causation. Emptiness defined the necessary precondition of fullness. The governing logic was that of war: *shi* was the excess of a body occupied by foreign intruders, *xu* the depletion of inner strength that invited intrusion.[100] The former corresponded to a surfeit of *xieqi*, noxious breaths from without; the latter, the lack of inner vitality. The *Suwen* succinctly summarized: "*Shi* is when *qi* comes in, *xu* is when *qi* goes out."[101]

This wasn't always the case, to be sure. "To reduce what is excessive, and to supplement insufficiency" (*sun youyu bu buzu*) was, Laozi taught, the Way of Heaven;[102] and this principle of compensation framed the meaning of acupuncture. Whereas bloodletting concentrated on excess, needling redressed tilts in both directions: it dispersed excess (*xie youyu*), but also supplemented insufficiency (*bu buzu*).[103] More generally, *xu* and *shi* sometimes just signaled relative imbalances in internal power and were synonymous with deficiency (*buzu*) and superfluity (*youyu*), falling short (*buji*) and going past (*guo*). A depletion (*xu*) of the kidneys, for instance, might result in the pathological ascendancy (*shi*) of the spleen. Damaged circulation following a blow might also cause a local *shi* congestion.

However, to the extent that Chinese physicians conceived of something more than relative or localized imbalance, to the extent that they imagined genuine excess, they tended to appeal to the model of alien influences — of wind and cold and other evils streaming in from without. If the plethoric fullness of the Greeks arose within the body, the fullness of *shi* highlighted the menaces of the surrounding world.

The presumably older guidelines for needling summarized in *Lingshu* treatise 1 are historically suggestive: "If empty (*xu*) then fill (*shi*) it; if replete (*man*), then flush it; if old, then remove it; if noxious breaths [from without] dominate, then empty (*xu*) them."[104]

Here we have not two but four principles of treatment, corresponding to four pathological states. The first compensates for emptiness, the others rectify three different kinds of fullness. Classical *xushi* analysis would subsequently obliterate the distinctions among the three kinds of fullness, and subsume them all under the single rubric of *shi*. And in doing so it would downplay the two pathologies paralleling those treated by Western phlebotomy, namely, repletion (arising presumably within the body) and the lingering of old stagnant substances. By defining *shi* as the influx of noxious breaths from without, classical medicine turned away from excesses native to the body and highlighted the paradigm of invasive occupation.

Let me be clear. There was nothing novel about fears of alien intrusion. Dread of demonic attack went back to Shang times, and remained strong in popular belief throughout Chinese history. The paradigm promoted by the scholarly medicine of the Han dynasty, however, departed from this tradition in two notable respects: first, it banished demons and evil spirits and identified intruders almost exclusively with the meteorological elements of wind and cold, heat, dampness, and dryness; and second, it made the harmfulness of these elements contingent on internal weakness. The latter was the prime innovation of *xushi* theory, the defining development in the formation of the classical Chinese understanding of sickness and the body.

Winds typically swept in through flaccid pores (a mark of depletion), then burrowed deeper — into the *mo*, then into the flesh, and finally into the organs and bones. But not everyone became a victim. Such evils could intrude only into depleted bodies.[105] The theory of *xu* and *shi* declared the priority of vulnerability, which is to say, emptiness. The *Lingshu* asseverated: "If wind, rain, cold or heat don't encounter a depletion [of bodily vitality], their *xieqi* alone can't harm people. When one unexpectedly experiences a windstorm or rainstorm and doesn't become ill, the reason must be that there is no depletion, and the *xieqi* alone can't harm people. Only when a depleting wind encounters a depletion within the body can [the wind] possess the body."[106] In a body brimming with vitality, there simply wasn't room for noxious influences to enter.

Greek and Chinese medicine thus evolved similarly in this sense: both came to stress the primacy of the body's inner state. Seeds of disease, gashes and bruises, violent winds, and cold all might harm and kill; but they were still secondary concerns. They really endangered only those predisposed toward sickness, just harmed the already sick. For the phlebotomist, pestilence and wounds festered only in bodies burdened by overeating and

222

indolence, bodies full of corrupting residues; for the acupuncturist, it was the emptiness of squandered vitality which invited the invasions of wind and cold. Bloodletting and acupuncture, in other words, both underlined the tendency of human beings to make themselves sick, but they diverged in their conceptions of dissolution.

Putrefaction, a phenomenon scarcely mentioned in acupuncture, haunted the phlebotomist's imagination of the body. Sickness was especially corruption. Blood was the substance of healthy flesh, but accumulating in excess, as unused residues in lethargic, indulged bodies, it fueled fevers and inflammations, hardened into monstrous growths, putrefied into pustulent ulcers. Whence the need for constant vigilance over incipient plethoras. Whence the need for prophylactic bleeding.

Disquiet in China revolved, contrarily, around dissipation and dispersal. Zhuangzi's famous aphorism equated life with the concentration of breath (qi) ("Qi gathered together is life; qi dispersed is death"[107]), and in late-Warring States and early Han times there emerged an exquisite sensitivity to how, in unguarded moments, life literally slipped away. Proponents of *yangsheng*, or the cultivation of life, brooded above all over the loss of precious essences in sexual abandon. But they also sensed vitality escaping from all the orifices. It flowed out of the eyes as one lingered on beautiful sights, and from the ears as one lost oneself to rapturous harmonies. The orifices were "the windows of the vital spirit," and sights and sounds drew this spirit outward, emptying the body, inviting affliction.[108]

This was desire — the streaming of life energy toward the desired object. Literally, as well as figuratively, desire entailed loss of self; lapses in self-possession and the depletion of vitality were but alternate faces of the same sickness. Conversely, somatic integrity and emotional self-mastery coalesced in health. As the philosopher Han Fei (d. 233 B.C.E.) concluded: "When the spirit does not flow outward, then the body is complete. When the body is complete, it is called powerful (*de*). Powerful refers to self-possessed (*zide*)."[109]

Though to us the men in figures 22 and 23 may look over-weight — models, we are almost tempted to say, of what the body should *not* be like — what their physiques in fact display is the promise of proper regimen. They are demonstrating exercises for *yangsheng*, the cultivation of life. We must see not flabby middle-age paunch here, but an ocean of vitality accumulated in the lower abdomen. Looking back to our very first picture (figure 1), we notice in the acupuncture man, too, the suggestion of relaxed capacious plenitude.

To be sure, the quietistic accumulation evoked by the sitting yogi wasn't the only ideal. Hua Tuo urged that "The body desires to exert itself (*laodong*)" and promoted exercises imitating the movements of animals. But the accent in this case fell on stimu-lating flow, and on shaping a pliant body. *Daoyin* was "the art of making the joints flexible" (*liguan zhi shu*). If self-contained full-ness was one goal, lithe fluidity was another. The stretchings and swayings that insured health could thus also be demonstrated by willowy women and by models whose robes billow as if blown by secret breezes (figures 24, 25, and 26). Disciplining the self nei-ther required, nor implied, the muscularity of the Vesalian man.

Exercise, in the Greek context, was virtually synonymous with strenuous labor (*ponos*). Remarks Galen, "The term [*ponos*] seems to me to have the same significance as exercise." And again, "In the care of health, work should come first." Exercise and work gave tone to the body and spurred the elimination of wastes; it worked, that is, against the drift toward plethoric excess.[110]

Unlike their Chinese counterparts, who worried about pores as avenues of intrusion, Greek doctors conceived them chiefly as

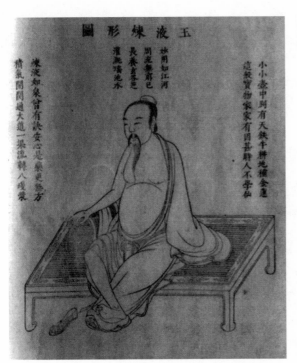
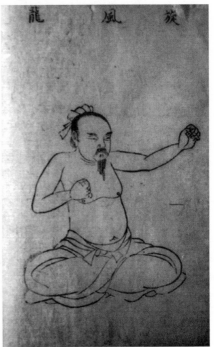

Figure 22. *Xingming zhi*, Shanghai Medical University.
Figure 23. *Jinshen jiyao*, Shanghai Medical University.

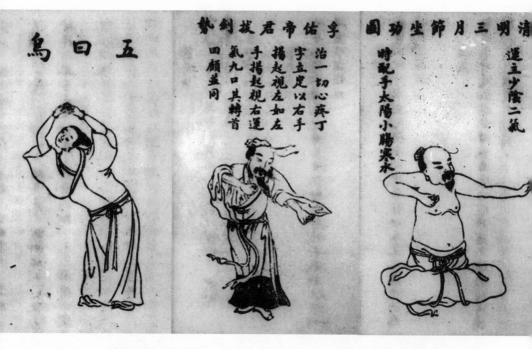

Figures 24–26. *Wuqin wugong tushuo* and *Zhuxian daoyin tu*, Shanghai Library.

paths of excretion, openings for expulsing superfluities. Their worries revolved around the evils of retention, rather than on the perils of invasion. Hence Galen's stress on menstrual regularity. It was essential, he held, that "the female sex, who stay indoors, neither engaging in strenuous labor nor exposing themselves to direct sunlight — both factors conducive to the development of plethos — should have a natural remedy by which it is released."[111] Menstruation was nature's substitute for the active male life.[112] Similarly, Aristotle observed that women accustomed to a life of hard work (ponētikos bios) found delivery easy: "The reason is that the effort of working uses up the residues, whereas sedentary women have a great deal of such matter in their bodies owing to the absence of effort, as well as to the cessation of the menstrual discharges during gestation, and they find the pains of delivery severe. Hard work, on the other hand, gives the breath exercise (ho de ponos gymnazei to pneuma)."[113]

Rather than quiet accumulation or breezy flexibility, Greek exercise promoted an articulated physique free of excess and a spirit tempered by strenuous effort. Vital breath was not something to be conserved and stored, but vigorously worked, through exertion of the will.

Underlying the split between bloodletting and acupuncture, then, was the difference between fears of corruption and fears of dissipation, between fears of retention and fears of loss. Whereas Greek medicine emphasized the benefits of menstruation, nosebleeds, and hemorrhoids as ways to forestall or relieve excess, Chinese physicians saw little good in nosebleeds and hemorrhoids; they simply tried to stop them. And though they recognized the need for regular menses, they treated lack of menstrual bleeding not so much as dangerous suppression, as a potential cause of sickness, but rather as a sign of exhausted blood, a consequence of prior depletion.[114]

Similar differences opposed views of intercourse. Sexual inactivity in women, Galen opined, and the resulting retention of the female seed, could induce more vicious harm even than the suppression of menstrual discharge. It could, for instance, cause a woman to become hysterical and suffocate. And while some men were admittedly weakened by excessive intercourse, others, "if they don't have regular sexual relations, feel heavy in the head, become nauseated and feverish, have a poor appetite and bad digestion." Even the Cynic philosopher Diogenes, "known to have been the most self-controlled of all people... indulged in sexual relations, since he wanted to get rid of the inconvenience caused by the retention of sperm."[115]

Ties between sex and sickness stirred anxieties in China as well; but these anxieties didn't revolve around pent-up seeds. Neither doctors nor yogic athletes promoted the need for prophylactic release. On the contrary. Their apprehensions circled obsessively around seed loss. They worried about too much intercourse, not its lack. Life was a finite resource, either wisely conserved to last over many healthy years, or recklessly, prematurely exhausted. Seeds were the purest concentrations of that life, and every drop lost meant a narrowing of vital possibilities. This is why adepts of the sexual discipline of *fangshu* so scrupulously studied techniques for retaining and "returning" the semen in intercourse.[116]

A pathology of corruption versus a pathology of dissipation. Apprehensions about retention and excess versus the dread of loss and lack. In probing the motivations of bloodletting and acupuncture, we have uncovered some provocative contrasts. As always, the contrasts are relative: doctors in China certainly recognized problems of excess, and their Greek counterparts didn't ignore sicknesses of depletion. Overall, however, intuitions of human frailty in the two traditions drew on opposing fears.

228

Let me return to a theme alluded to at the chapter's start, namely, the relationship of blood to breath.

Phlebotomy and acupuncture would seem to differ most plainly in this: the former treated blood, the latter, *qi*, breath. But this characterization is imprecise. In Chinese medicine, blood and *qi* were essentially the same. Doctors did, to be sure, occasionally spotlight distinctions. Blood had form, for instance, while *qi* was formless; the former was constructive, making up the substance of the body, the latter was protective, warding off alien pathogens. Diagnostically, slippery *mo* indicated more blood than *qi*, a rough *mo* bespoke the reverse. Therapeutically, when bloodletting was still practiced, some ailments required the healer to "Let blood, but no *qi*," while for others one had to "Let *qi*, but no blood." But all these represented differences in aspect, not essence. Ultimately, blood and *qi* were complementary facets of a unique vitality, its yin and yang manifestations.[117]

Crisper dichotomies tended to oppose blood and *pneuma* in Greek thought. For the presocratic Diogenes, the divide between air and blood thus underlay the contrast between pleasure and pain.[118] In Aristotle's embryology, the female blood provided the material substance of the body, while *pneuma* from the male sperm articulated the body's form.[119] Although ancient ideas of *pneuma* underwent complex change, and although blood and *pneuma* remained entwined in many respects, we can discern nonetheless a gradual trend toward polarization, whereby blood became identified with the passive, corruptible materiality of the body, while *pneuma* became linked to the activities and essence of the soul.[120] Suggestively, Chinese doctors supposed vitality to flow in a single network of channels, the *mo*, whereas Greek medicine soon segregated blood and *pneuma* into separate conduits: veins carried mostly blood and sustained such "vegetative" functions as nutrition and growth, while nerves, filled uniquely with *pneuma*, carried sensation and will.[121] Blood borne by the veins became flesh; but it was *pneuma* streaming from the brain and through the nerves which transformed plantlike flesh into muscle, an *organon psychichon*, an instrument of the soul.[122]

Then there were the arteries, conduits of a third kind, from whose motions doctors divined a patient's past, present, and future life. The claims of evacuation allow us now to reconsider such divinations in a new light; reconsider, too, why Greek diagnosticians couldn't rest content with mere beats and pauses — why they had to track the artery in its contractions and dilations.

Living people are warm, corpses are cold, and as humans age their bodies become cooler, easily chilled. Since Plato's *Timaeus*, at least, Greek reflections on vitality saw special significance in the ties between life and warmth.[123] Preserving life required stoking a sort of internal physiological fire, maintaining what Aristotle termed innate heat. Food provided the essential fuel; without it, the fire would die. For the well-nourished, however, the more pressing threat was the opposite. Until one grew old and the innate heat waned, a person needed constant refrigeration to keep from burning up.[124] This was one reason why one had to breathe to live. As breath was sucked in and filled the lungs, it cooled and counterbalanced the heat of the inborn fire. As breath was expelled, it drew out the hot, smoky residues.

It was precisely this same cycle of cooling and elimination that also defined the use of the pulse. On this, physicians as diverse as Erasistratus, Asclepiades, and Galen concurred: the purpose of pulsation was to regulate the innate heat.[125] If the pulse provided a sensitive gauge of human life, it was partly because it played, itself, a key role in safeguarding that life.

Pulse motions resembled the movements of the thorax. Greek physicians imagined small pores in the arterial wall, which functioned like the nose and mouth of the respiratory system. Diastole corresponded to the expansion of the thorax: both motions drew in air from the outside and cooled the body. Arterial systole and the fall of the chest in exhalation, on the other hand, both worked to expulse smoky residues, squeezing them out. The only differences, then, between respiration and pulsation were: (1) whereas the former cooled and cleansed the heart, the pulse performed these functions for the body as a whole; and (2) whereas breathing could be altered by the will — one could hold one's breath, for example, at least for a while — the arteries moved involuntarily.[126]

Physical exertion and fevers naturally increase the size and frequency of both respiratory movements and the pulse — these changes compensate for the increase in heat and residues. With regard to the pulse specifically, Galen noted that, in people who sleep after eating copiously, "the expansive beat of the pulse is faint, becoming both lower and slower; the contraction, on the other hand, increases in both ways, appearing both faster than before and reaching more deeply in."[127] This was because the digestive process drew the innate heat inward, and because the breakdown of food produced large quantities of superfluities that needed to be expelled. Systole was also accentuated in children, "for the working up of the humors is particularly great in them, on account of their growth. On the other hand, old people are found to have the contraction very slow and shallow, because it is sluggish and weak in concoction and does little to work up the humors, since it is unnecessary."[128]

Galen's instructions on positioning the fingers and pressing the artery were directed toward one goal: the clear grasp of the systole.[129] We now see why. The artery's two motions had distinct and separate implications.[130] If one couldn't feel the systole one remained deaf to at least half of the pulse's message. One couldn't inspect that function whose faltering was responsible for so many calamities. One couldn't judge the elimination of superfluities.

CHAPTER SIX

Wind and Self

There was much rain in Thasos about the time of the autumnal equinox and during the season of the Pleiads. It fell gently and continuously and the wind was from the south. During the winter, the wind blew mostly from the south; winds from the north were few and the weather was dry. On the whole the winter was like springtime; but the spring was cold with southerly winds and there was little rain. The summer was for the most part cloudy but there was no rain. The Etesian winds were few and light and blew at scattered intervals.[1]

These lines open the Hippocratic journal, *Epidemics* 1. We imagine them easily in a farmer's diary, or a seafarer's log. They wouldn't be strange as the start of some lyric tale. Oddly, it is hardest to read them for what they were, as medical remarks on the signs of imminent suffering. We rarely think of wind, now, when we think of sickness. Southerly breezes and light Etesian winds no longer count among life's fundamental forces.

Yet wind was once an constant concern. The keen sense of its sway over what and when and how afflictions afflict, so striking in *Epidemics* 1, reappears in many Hippocratic writings — in *Epidemics* 3, and *Aphorisms*, and *Airs, Waters, Places*, and in the treatises *On Breaths*, *On Humors*, *On Regimen*, and *On the Sacred Disease*.[2]

A damp winter with southerly breezes followed by a dry spring with northerly winds induces miscarriages, dysentery, dry ophthalmia, and catarrhs. On the other hand, "If the summer is dry with northerly winds, and the autumn wet with wind in the south, the winter brings a danger of headaches and gangrene of the brain." Epileptic seizures are apt to occur "at any change of wind, especially when it is southerly."[3] It is doubtless with such lessons in mind that *Airs, Waters, Places* cites, as the first two subjects that the aspiring doctor must master, "the effect of each of the seasons of the year" and "the warm and cold winds, both those common to every country and those peculiar to a particular locality."[4] No one could pretend to know the body who didn't know the winds.

Nor was this view unique to the Greeks. In the classics of Chinese medicine, winds (*feng*) cause chills and headaches, vomiting and cramps, dizziness and numbness, loss of speech. And that is but the beginning. "Wounded by wind" (*shangfeng*), a person burns with fever. "Struck by wind" (*zhongfeng*), another drops suddenly senseless. Winds can madden, even kill. Where now we scarcely blame wind for any afflictions, Chinese doctors traditionally suspected its ravages in nearly all. "Wind is the chief of the hundred diseases," the *Neijing* declared. And again, "The hundred diseases arise from wind."[5]

The imagination of winds is virtually invisible in the historiography of medicine. Indices of the older grand surveys — such as those of Singer and Underwood, Neuberger, Garrison, Castiglione, Sigerist, Ackerknecht, Bass, and Gordon — flag trifles like wigs and wintergreen oil, window tax, and Wong, the collector of proverbs; but none lists wind.[6] And while more recent cultural historians have traced the vagaries of mind and body, food and body, the gendered body, and the body politic, few have even noticed the existence, much less pondered the meaning, of the ties binding the body to wind.[7]

Yet for many in the past these ties seemed unimaginably potent and profound. Winds sculpted the shape and possibilities of the body, molded desires and dispositions, infused a person's entire being. People who live in districts exposed to northerly winds, *Airs, Waters, Places* reports, are "sturdy and lean, tend to constipation, their bowels being intractable but their chests will move easily.... Such men eat with good appetites but they drink little. ... Characters are fierce rather than tame." By contrast, those living in areas exposed to winds from the quarter between northeast and south-east, "have loud and clear voices, and ... are of better temperament and intelligence than those exposed to the north."[8] Plato likewise cites the diversity of winds as a major reason why "some places produce better men and others worse," and why different laws have to be crafted for each locality. For local winds, along with the local earth and food, "not only affect the bodies of men for good or evil, but also produce these results in their souls."[9]

Parallel beliefs informed the Chinese term for the local customs, *fengsu*. According to the *Hanshu*, the compound *fengsu* contained the word *feng*, wind, because people's natures are literally inspired by the air that they breathe: "Though human nature is framed by the five constancies, some peoples are more rigid, others more flexible, some are relaxed, others tense, and their voices differ in pitch. All these qualities depend on the windy breath (*fengqi*) of the region. This is why the term for customs (*fengsu*) invokes the notion of wind (*feng*)."[10]

Geography was destiny, and wind the instrument of fate. In *fengshui*, the art of "wind and water," diviners diagnosed the flow of breaths in each locality and sought out the best sites for the living to live and the dead to rest. Suggestively, they called these sites *xue*, holes or caverns — a name that recalled associations between winds and the earth's hollows[11] and that was also identical to what acupuncturists called the sites they needled to channel the flow of *qi*. In English the acupuncture sites mapping the body in figure 2 are blandly called "points." The original term *xue*, however, conjured a vision of the body in which winds streamed in and out of strategic orifices in the skin, just as winds blew in and out of the caverns of the earth.

These remarks point toward a crucial aspect of the ties between body and wind: in both Chinese and Greek antiquity the winds blowing *around* the body were often presumed to be related to the breaths sustaining the life *within*. Hiraoka Teikichi, Akatsuka Tadashi, and others have thus pointed out how the discourse of *qi* which emerged in Warring States times had roots in the far more ancient tradition of meditations on wind.[12] Even in Han times, indeed, *feng* and *qi* were frequently interchangeable. "Wind is *qi*" (*fu feng zhe, qi ye*) glossed Wang Chong; and the *Neijing*, conversely, explained that, "What is meant by healthy *qi* (*zhengqi*) is healthy wind" (*zhengfeng*)."[13] In classical Greek, the intimacy between wind and breath appears even more plainly: the same term, *pneuma*, could evoke both. When the chorus chants about Antigone, "Yet from the same winds still / These blasts of soul hold her," it speaks simultaneously of the external winds driving destinies and the swerves of inner passion.[14]

In this way, meditations on human life were once inseparable from meditations on wind. But we tend to forget this now: a profound oblivion separates the present from the past, and the exquisite ancient sensitivity to wind has come to seem a strange and distant dream. We no longer possess a ready feel for the experience of being that it mirrors. Querying the imagination of winds in antiquity we can be sure only of this: the history of the body is ultimately a history of ways of inhabiting the world.

What sort of world was it in which bodies were so influenced by wind? And how did the belief in wind's sway, once shared by Greek and Chinese doctors alike, relate to the divergent conceptions of the body that evolved in Greek and Chinese medicine? These are broad issues that frame the final chapter of our inquiry.

What is Wind?

Of the various enigmas surrounding wind, that of its identity is perhaps the most puzzling. We hear of winds causing seizures, paralysis, and madness, we are told of how they shape bodies and minds, and we cannot but wonder: What is wind? Often, the winds blowing in ancient texts sound quite unlike the winds that we know now.

"Will the wind come from the east?" "Will the wind come the west?" "Will destructive wind arise?" "Will wind bring rain tomorrow?" Such questions recur in the earliest Chinese inscriptions — the queries of Shang diviners dating as far back as the thirteenth century B.C.E. The reference to rain hints at one motivating interest: wind is weather, and weather ultimately wind. Linguists tell us that the English word "weather" derives from the Indo-Germanic root *we*, "to blow." Winds may bring nourishing showers to the fields, or sweep in bitter frost, they may stir up the storms that make hunting dangerous, or stay still, and cause sweltering drought. Rain, frost, storms, and drought can decide famine or prosperity for millions, even today. In the past, when life hung even more precariously on weather-sensitive endeavors like farming, hunting, and fishing, it seems only natural that wind should inspire awe.

Awe is the exact term. Shang winds were not mere move-

237

ments of air, but divine presences. Sacrifices called them forth or sought their retreat. And the direction from which they blew was crucial: the cardinal directions staked out distinct spiritual abodes imbued with distinct powers, and the winds blowing out of them ruled the metamorphoses of the world.[15] They shifted direction, and abundant game became sparse; shifted again, and a losing battle turned to victory.

Shang kings had to be ever alert to this dynamic. "Should the king begin his tour in the south?" the oracles query. "Should the king hunt to the east?" Whether it be royal tours of the kingdom or the hunting of game, the fate of all endeavors revolved around timely orientation. "Should the king begin his tour in the north?" "Will the king encounter great wind in the hunt today?" Hunting in the west when one should be hunting in the east was at best fruitless, at worst fatal. On the other hand, of one king who presumably heeded the oracles we learn: "Today, the king hunted in the east, and indeed captured three pigs."[16]

Later ages came to speak rather less of gods, but a sense of amazement remained. Spring breezes blew, and suddenly insects began to stir, horses and cows were seized by the urge to mate.[17] The *Huainanzi* marveled at wind's workings, its scale and effortless ease:

> When the spring wind arrives, tender rains fall, nurturing the myriad things.... Grasses and trees burst forth and flower, and birds and animals reproduce. All of this is accomplished, and yet we don't see the effort. Autumn wind brings frost, retreat, decline.... The grasses and trees retrench to their roots, fish and turtles crowd back into the deep. All is reduced to formless desolation; yet we don't see the effort.[18]

238

One day we revel in a world of brilliant colors and soft abundance, the next day we turn to face gray barren hardness. Here is a friend whom just last year we saw laughing, happy, vigorous; now we see only the shadow of a person, emaciated, drawn, on the verge of death. How do such things happen? Many sought the secret in wind.

Winds foreshadowed change, exemplified change, caused change, *were* change. They presaged the waxing and waning of imperial charisma,[19] warned of imminent wars and famines. Among the works of He Xiu, the great Han-dynasty authority on the *Spring and Autumn Annals*, was a commentary on a treatise of *fengzhan*, wind divination;[20] and the historian Sima Qian reports how the diviner Wei Xian interpreted the winds at dawn of the first day of the new year:

> If wind comes from the south, there will be great drought. If it comes from the southwest, a minor drought. If it comes from the west, there will be military uprisings. If it comes from the northwest, the soybeans will ripen well, rains will be few, and armies will move. If it comes from the north, the harvest will be average. If it comes from the northeast, there will an exceptional harvest. If it comes from the east, there will be floods. If it comes from the southeast, there will be epidemics among the people, and the harvest will be bad....[21]

Winds thus held the key to rich harvests and fatal famines, floods and epidemics, war and peace. And more: Wang Chong recounts how contemporaries tracked their direction and timing in order to forecast the changing moods of the populace, and even to foretell individual fortunes.[22]

Riddles of mutability were always central to wind's fascination. In Greek tragedy, winds regularly bore the vagaries of luck, as the breath of immortal gods altering mortal fate. "Fools!" teaches Euripides' Theseus, "Be instructed in the ills of man."

> Struggles make up our life. Good fortune comes
> Swiftly to some, to some hereafter; others
> Enjoy it now. Its god luxuriates.
> Not only is he honored by the hapless
> In hope of better days, but lucky ones
> Exalt him too, fearing to lose the wind.[23]

Those enjoying smooth sailing are nervous about losing the wind, while the less lucky hope to catch it. For both, the pneumatic character of life makes all happiness fragile, all peace insecure. At any moment a "veering change of wind" may turn fortune into misfortune.[24]

To Theseus' query about how war could arise between two longstanding allies, Oedipus replies,

> Most gentle son of Aegeus! The immortal
> Gods alone have neither age nor death!
> All other things almighty Time disquiets.
> Earth wastes away; distrust is born.
> And imperceptibly the wind shifts
> Between a man and his friend, or between two cities.
> For some men soon, for others in later time,
> Their pleasure sickens; or love comes again.[25]

And imperceptibly the wind shifts. Lovers awaken one morning to discover their ardor inexplicably cooled. Somehow, before they realize it, close friends become twisted with distrust. Rains plentiful for years abruptly dry up. Overnight, a peaceful people thirst for blood. Meditations on the obscure origins of such changes kept returning to the secret of wind's turns.

The shifts in wind here — between allied cities, between friends and lovers — are of course metaphorical. To appreciate the full force of the metaphor, however, we must reenter a world in which winds were experienced as immanent powers, vivid presences. By sending fair breezes, by blowing gales, by stopping wind altogether, the gods could transport mariners swiftly home, or drown them, or make them drift aimlessly — as the *Odyssey* reminds us.

Aiolus, warden of the winds, supplies Odysseus for his journey home with a huge sack full of storm winds. Odysseus' men suspect that the sack contains gold and silver, and untie it, releasing a hurricane that sweeps them far off course.[26] The men were perhaps foolish, but in a way they weren't far wrong: the sack did contain a treasure, and for sailors the most valuable — wind, fortune itself.

"Will the wind come from the east?" Shang shamans asked. "Will the wind come the west?" That summer, *Epidemics* 1 observes, the Etesian winds were few and light and blew at scattered intervals. The poets who likened the swerve of passions to the veering of winds lived alongside sailors whose very lives turned with the wind, alongside diviners and physicians who believed that winds brought fortune and misfortune, health and sickness.

We asked about the sources of the medical preoccupation with wind. We find hints of an answer in the claims of change. On the one hand, the study of sickness is the study of altered states, on the other, "Wind," as Chinese commentaries summed up, "is transformation" (*feng hua ye*). Herodotus observes that Egyptians are healthy because their seasons don't change. "For people are most likely to be seized with maladies during changes; changes of anything, but especially of the seasons."[27]

241

The history of wind and the body is the history of the relationship between change and human being.

Wind and Breath

How does one lead a population to love the good and to follow the path of virtue? People can be unpredictable. One week they are seized by a rage for revolution, the following week they resist even the most modest reforms. One year they reject old values because they are old, a decade later, they embrace old values because they are old. All rulers must solve the riddle of such turns.

> Ji Kangzi asked Confucius about government, saying, "What would you think if, in order to move closer to those who possess the Way, I were to kill those who did not follow the Way?"
>
> Confucius answered, "In administering your government, what need is there for you to kill? Just desire good yourself and the common people will be good. The gentleman's virtue is like the wind; the virtue of the common people is like grass. The wind sweeps over the grass, and the grass is sure to bend."[28]

The *Huainanzi* wondered at the effortlessness of seasonal change, at how winds could dress the entire earth in dazzling hues or turn it drab brown and gray, all with no trace of exertion. Confucius's vision of government by virtue reflected analogous instincts about change in the human heart, about what makes people turn from evil to good. It wasn't brute force or fear. A more spiritual, that is, more breathlike logic ruled the heart. Governing was less a matter of coercing or intimidating than of swaying, gently and indirectly.

In much the way that music moves the heart. The *Classic of Odes*, the oldest collection of Chinese poetry, opens with a section called *Guofeng*, "Airs of the States." Here was another major

242

sense of *feng*: *feng* were songs, airs. Ritual dance was ruled by the eight tones and eight airs (*bafeng*). Music encompassed the "five notes, six pitch-pipes, seven tones, eight airs, and nine songs."[29]

Rulers knew a people by the songs they sang. When Prince Ji Zha of Wu visited Sun Muzi he asked the latter's singers to perform songs from each of the various states. Whereas he found the airs of Zheng too refined and prophesied that Zheng would soon perish, he judged the songs of Qi to be "great airs" (*dafeng*), giving voice to a state with unfathomable possibilities.[30] Ji Zha presumably discerned in the airs of the various states the feelings and disposition of the people who sang them. The *Lüshi chunqiu* observed, "One hears the music [of a state] and knows its customs (*feng*). By examining this *feng* one knows the aspirations (*zhi*) [of the people], and by scrutinizing these aspirations, one knows their virtue — whether it is rising or declining, whether [the people are] wise or foolish, sagely or petty. All this is manifest in the music and cannot be hidden."[31]

Alternatively we might translate: "One hears the music of a state and knows its mood (*feng*)." Airs, mood, customs all expressed the spirit of a place. All arose from local winds.

Airs were also *feng* because they influenced and transformed, because they altered feelings and comportment. Here again, the key was indirection: "By airs (*feng*) superiors transform their inferiors, and by airs inferiors satirize their superiors. The principal thing lies in their style, and reproof is cunningly insinuated. They can be spoken without giving offense, and yet hearing them suffices to make people circumspect in their behavior. This is why they are called *feng*."[32]

The *Guofeng* were first compiled, the Great Preface to the *Odes* relates, because "the kingly way had declined, and propriety and righteousness had been abandoned."[33] Appropriate airs were collected to save the state by reorienting attitudes, swaying behavior. The Lesser Preface adds that "Airs originated as a means for transforming (*feng*) the empire and regulating the relations between husband and wife." For modifying mores (*yifeng yisu*), Confucius held, nothing surpasses music.[34]

It was Zhuangzi, though, in his meditations on "the music of heaven," who offered perhaps the most eloquent summary of the interplay between wind, music, feeling, and human identity:

> The Great Clod (the earth) belches out breath and its name is wind. So long as it doesn't come forth, nothing happens. But when it does, then ten thousand hollows begin crying wildly. Can't you hear them, long drawn out? In the mountain forests that lash and sway, there are huge trees a thousand spans around with hollows and openings like noses, like mouths, like ears, like jugs, like cups, like rifts, like ruts. They roar like waves, whistle like arrows, screech, gasp, cry, wail, moan, and howl, and those in the lead calling out yeee!, and those behind calling out yuuu! In a gentle breeze they answer faintly, but in a full gale the chorus is gigantic. And when the fierce wind has passed on, then all the hollows are empty again.

Zhuangzi termed this symphony of wind rushing through the hollows "the music of the earth." But this earthly music echoed "the music of heaven," the silent music of the pneumatic self:

> Pleasure and anger, sorrow and joy, anxiety and regret, fickleness and fear, impulsiveness and extravagance, indulgence and lewdness, come to us like music from the hollows or like mushrooms from damp. Day and night they alternate within us but we don't know where they come from....
>
> Without them (the feelings mentioned above) there would not be I. And without me who will experience them? They are right near by. But we don't know who causes them.[35]

The winds of moral suasion, the airs that rectify the heart, and now the heavenly music of gaiety and sadness. All these bespeak a fluid, ethereal existence in a fluid, ethereal world. A living being is but a temporary concentration of breath (*qi*), death merely the scattering of this breath.[36] There is an I, Zhuangzi assures us, a self. But this self is neither a shining Orphic soul imprisoned in the darkness of matter, nor an immaterial mind set against a material body. Anchored in neither reason nor will, it is a self without essence, the site of moods and impulses whose origins are beyond reckoning, a self in which thoughts and feelings arise spontaneously, of themselves, like the winds whistling through the earth's hollows.

Early Greek writers, too, allude to the inseparability of breath and being. Homeric heroes filled with surging passion and energy "breathe *menos*";[37] in Aeschylus, warriors at war "breathe Ares."

To an extent, these express familiar, everyday observations: we know the rough panting of those pushed to extraordinary exertions, the spasmodic heaving of people overwhelmed by emotion. Ruth Padel, however, has astutely observed the ambiguity of these phrases — how "often it is impossible for a listener to know which way the breath of emotion is flowing, and therefore where its source is."

> When Aeschylus speaks of a man "breathing Ares," we could take it as "breathing out a fighting rage," and imagine that the warrior's breath breathed *out* in battle "is" the war-god. Later in the same play Cassandra sees the house breathing *phobon* ("bloodshed").

> But in another play "breaths of Ares" appear as if they came from god *into* people, blasting the city, urging besiegers on. Someone is "entheos" (possessed) with (or by) Ares. Given Greek resonances of

possession as an incoming divine breath, this suggests that Ares breathes *into* the warrior.[38]

The word *pneuma*, in classical drama, refers more often to wind than to breath. "Winter comes by sharp winds," chants the chorus in Aeschylus' *Suppliant Maidens*. "The wind's course veers," says Euripides' Creusa.[39] But almost always, the winds evoked in this way are entwined with the course of human lives, with shifts of fortune, with people's changing thoughts, the flow of feelings. Padel notes, "When his (Euripides's) chorus praises Electra for a pious change in attitude, it says, 'Your thought has veered again to the breeze.' Peleus thinks Menelaus should have ignored Helen's departure: 'But not that way did you set your thought to the wind.' Menelaus was the helmsman of his thought, but there were real winds outside him."[40]

This is perhaps the most striking trait of the early discourse on winds — the remarkable looseness of what now seem like firm boundaries, the blurriness of the divide separating outer flux and inner vitality, winds from breath.

But these are the words of poets and philosophers. We would expect physicians to be more rigorous. And in fact, the Hippocratic treatise *On Breaths* does draw distinctions: *pneuma* inside the body is called breath (*physa*); outside the body it is called air (*aēr*); and the flow of this air is wind (*anemos*). But the very point of this work is to affirm the unity of outer and inner *pneuma*, of wind and breath, and to accuse disruptions in its flow as the cause of all disease. At the same time that it describes the afflictions arising from blocked breath within the body, the work waxes eloquent about how *pneuma* fills heaven and earth, brings summer and winter, guides the course even of the sun and the stars.[41]

Admittedly, some have judged *On Breaths* a sophistical work, more notable for rhetorical flourish than medical insight; it may not be thought the best of evidence.[42] Yet consider *On the Sacred Disease*, one of the most admired of Hippocratic treatises. It rejects supernatural causation, argues from postmortem dissections, and comes as close as any Hippocratic work to the long-influential notion of nerves filled with *pneuma*. Air drawn in through the mouth and nose, the treatise relates, first flows to the brain and induces intelligence; flowing from the brain through hollow veins, it mediates the movement of the limbs. This is why when phlegm obstructs air's passage through the veins a person may lose the power of speech or suffer convulsions.[43] Epileptic seizures, popularly attributed to divine possession, really arise from blocked air.

The term used here for obstructed breath is actually not *pneuma* but *aēr* — a small detail, but noteworthy because the same histories that tout the pioneering role of the *Sacred Disease* in the development of Greek pneumatism regularly slight the *pneumata* that the treatise itself actually calls *pneumata*. They rarely dwell on the fact that the treatise is as concerned with the influence of wind as with the flow of inner breath.

Blocked air accounts only for the immediate symptoms. Ultimately, epilepsy and other diseases are caused by "matters going in and out of the body, cold, sun, and the ever changing restless winds." Seizures thus most often occur

> when the wind is southerly; less when it is northerly, less still when it is in any other quarter; for the south and north winds are the strongest of the winds and the most opposed in direction and in influence.
>
> The north wind precipitates the moisture in the air so that the cloudy and damp elements are separated out leaving the atmosphere clear and bright. It treats similarly all the other vapors which arise from the sea or form other stretches of water, distilling out from them the damp and dark elements. It does the same for human beings and it is therefore the healthiest wind.

247

The south wind has just the opposite effect. It starts by vaporizing the precipitated moisture because it does not generally blow very hard at first. The calm period occurs because the wind cannot immediately absorb the moisture in the air which was previously dense and congealed, but loosens it in time. The south wind has the same effect on the earth, the sea, rivers, springs, wells and everything that grows or contains moisture. In fact, everything contains moisture in a greater or lesser degree and thus all these things feel the effect of the south wind and become dark instead of bright, warm instead of cold, and moist instead of dry. Jars in the house or in the cellars which contain wine or any other liquid are influenced by the south wind and change their appearance. The south wind also makes the sun, moon and stars much dimmer than usual.

Seeing that such large and powerful bodies are overcome, and that the human body is made to feel changes of wind and undergo changes at that time, it follows that southerly winds relax the brain and make it flabby, relaxing the blood-vessels at the same time. Northerly winds, on the other hand, solidify the healthy part of the brain while any morbid part is separated out and forms a fluid layer around the outside.[44]

I quote this passage at length because it illustrates the two most salient features of how Greek doctors perceived wind. The first is the focus on northerly and southerly breezes. The great majority of the many remarks about winds in the *Sacred Disease*, *Epidemics* 1 and 3, and *Airs, Waters, Places* concern those blowing from the north or the south; we hear far less about other winds — those from the east or west, or directions in between. North and south winds are, we are told, the strongest and the most opposed in influence. So tight was their presumed tie that *On Humors* asserts the possibility of predicting from the prevailing diseases the arrival of north and south winds.[45]

248

This characteristic relates to a second feature of Greek pneumatic analysis, namely, its foundation in the dialectic of qualities.[46] North wind is cool and dry, south wind is warm and moist. Homer already calls the north wind *Aithrēgenetēs*, "creating clear sky": it drives away the clouds.[47] By contrast, the very term for south wind, *notos*, evokes moisture, *notis*.[48] The author of *Sacred Disease* is unequivocal about what these different qualities imply: north wind is healthful, south wind brings sickness.[49]

Northerly winds are healthy because they make the body drier, cooler, firmer; southerly winds induce flabbiness. The moisture-laden breezes from the south make the air hazy, dim the sun, the moon, the stars. They cloud even liquids stored in jars. Small wonder, then, that they should similarly affect the body, and not just the body, but also the mind. The author of *Airs, Waters, Places*, recall, believed that bracing cold made Europeans not only stronger and more virile than the moist and effeminate barbarians, but also smarter.

The opposition of northerly and southerly breezes, in other words, belonged to the skein of associations that linked the moist with the weak, the feminine, the flabby and the stupid, cloudiness, surfeit, putrefaction. The warm wet winds from the south were the winds that made barbarians soft and sickly; and they were the winds of pestilence.[50] Theophrastus, for his part, discerned the contrasting effects of dry and moist air in the intellectual disparity separating humans from animals: "Thought . . . is caused by pure and dry air; for a moist emanation inhibits the intelligence; for this reason thought is diminished in sleep, drunkenness, and surfeit. That moisture removes intelligence is indicated by the fact that other living creatures are inferior in intellect, for they breathe the air from the earth and take to themselves moister sustenance."[51] Humans are more intelligent because their heads are further removed from the moist earth, because they inspire drier air.

In Greek medicine, then, winds transformed not as some special, independent force, but by virtue of their dryness or moistness, warmth or cold. It was because all things were governed by the dialectics of dry and wet, hot and cold, that northerly and southerly breezes induced irresistible, thoroughgoing changes — in people, in the surrounding land and sea, in not just the human body, but even in "large and powerful bodies" like the sun, the moon, and the stars.

In the end, the fact that warmth and moisture happened to be borne by the south wind was incidental: the encounter was not between winds and bodies, but between their defining qualities — the immersion in something warm and wet, say, of something cooler and drier. Southerly winds made vision misty, clouded the mind, spread languor in the limbs. And they produced these effects not by directly invading the eyes or brain, but more circuitously: their humid warmth distended blood vessels and flesh, and caused moist vapors to rise and fill the head, bloat the body. Winds harmed by heating or cooling, drying or moistening. Though remarkable in the range of their influence, the hot, humid winds from the south were just one of several causes that made things go slack.

This scheme of winds and qualities continued, long after Hippocrates, to shape the imagination of bodily presence in the world. It explained, for instance, the prevalence in winter of catarrhs — the downflow of phlegm from the brain into the nose, throat, and mouth. For "Coldness doth compress the brain," observed Lazarus Rivière, "and strains forth the humor therein contained, as a sponge is squeezed by the hand. Such change is often in winter, and especially in sudden alteration of air: as when a southern wind hot and moist is turned into a north wind cold and dry."[52] It also remained basic to conceptions of local constitution. Northerners were robust, according to Jean Bodin (1530?–96), because "Winds flowing from the south are warm and damp; from the north cold and dry." Montesquieu (1689–1755) likewise opined that the opposition of the cold north and warm south divided strong, spirited warriors from feebler, sybaritic dispositions.[53]

Winds figured rather differently in Chinese medicine. For doctors in China, wind represented less a distant, exciting cause of disease, inciting imbalances within the body, than disease itself, an alien invader. It swept straight *into* the body's interior and harmed by intrusion. Attacking the skin, it might produce chills, headache, a slight fever; as it burrowed deeper, it wrought more intractable, more violent suffering. The winds of the four quarters, moreover, formed an indivisible set. Northerly and southerly breezes in Chinese medicine held no more sway than winds from the east or west, and winds from any direction could nurture or harm. Though wind sometimes attacked in tandem with cold, or heat, or moisture, it basically stood separate as an independent source of sickness. Winds were never grouped by their temperature or humidity. Wind was feared *as* wind.

Yet what could it mean, really, to fear wind as wind? Where did wind's threat lie if not in its coolness or warmth, moisture or dryness? The recurring images of attack and intrusion recall archaic fears of demonic fury, of thrashing possession by restless spirits. And this was almost certainly part of the sense of wind's menace in ancient China; the currents that harmed were called *xiefeng*, evil winds. One imagines roving malign influences.

However, the *Neijing* never actually speaks of demons in connection with wind. Nor does subsequent medical literature: Chao Yuanfang's influential nosology, the *Zhubing yuanhou lun* (610), opens with an extended survey of wind afflictions, and over a thousand years later the encyclopedic *Gujin tushu jicheng* begins its exposition of the causes of disease with no less than eight *juan* (more than seven hundred pages of the original edition) to disorders caused by wind — by far the longest section on any pathogen. From Han through Qing times, Chinese writings consistently assign a special, dominant role to wind in human suffering. But not because winds are gods. Whatever the popular or subliminal associations of wind with the world of spirits, formal medical treatises concentrated on a different danger.

Shang wind divinities could make one sick. This was one reason why Shang shamans performed sacrifices to appease them.[54] But this doesn't seem to have been a major motive: what made appeasement so urgent was rather wind's broader influence on crops, hunting, and government. As for sickness, the preponderance of Shang references blame the vengeance of unhappy ancestors.[55] Most fevers, headaches, and other ailments derived from ancestral curses. "Divining this tooth affliction. Should we hold a festival for Fuyi?" "Ringing in the ears. Should we sacrifice a hundred sheep to Ancestor Geng?" Diagnosis sought to uncover the disgruntled ancestor — whether it be Fuyi, Ancestor Geng, or someone other; prevention and treatment required rituals to dissolve the dissatisfactions of the dead.

By the Spring and Autumn era, we start to glimpse other emphases. Why do people fall ill? The physician Yi He (sixth century B.C.E.) ignored demonic attacks, but instead blamed six causes: the yin, the yang, wind, rain, darkness, and brightness. All these, he taught, are necessary to the world's working, but in excess, they harm. Much yin brings cold diseases, much yang, fevers; wind strikes the limbs, rain, the abdomen; darkness induces delusions, brightness, disorders of the mind.[56] Thus while Yi He recognized distinct dangers in wind, he didn't privilege its menace. As a cause of sickness wind was merely one among six.[57]

Only with the *Neijing* do we find it spotlighted, for the first time in history, as "the beginning of the hundred diseases." The extant evidence about Shang and Zhou medicine is sparse, of course, so by itself the argument from silence is weak. But there is another, stronger reason for supposing the novelty of the *Neijing*'s stress on wind. It concerns the very definition of wind's evil.

Not all winds bore harm. Wind etiology in the *Neijing* and in all subsequent medical literature turned on the divide opposing "proper" or "full" winds (*zhengfeng*; *shifeng*), on the one hand, against "evil" or "empty" winds (*xiefeng*; *xufeng*), on the other; opposing, that is, nurturing winds against harmful winds. Proper winds were essential to human health and, more generally, to cosmic order. At times, it is true, they could blow too strongly and cause sickness; but they didn't for all that cease to be proper. The maladies they induced were always minor, and people soon recovered from them, even without treatment.[58] All the serious assaults on the body and the mind were the work of evil winds.

The opposition of the proper and the evil had nothing to with qualities of air — with fresh, pure breezes, say, versus polluted breaths. Nor were good and evil assigned to fixed directions; neither northerly or southerly winds were full or empty in and of themselves. The crux of the matter lay, instead, in timing.

Proper, full winds were those that blew from the right direction in the right season: easterly winds in spring, southerly winds in summer, westerly winds in fall, northerly winds in winter. Evil, empty winds were those that deviated from this rule, that blew from the north in summer, say, or conversely, wafted up in winter from the south. They were evil because they contravened against an ideal order. Their intrusion was the intrusion of chaos.[59]

The etiology of wind was thus framed by a cosmic scheme. Wind's menace was that of time gone awry. Here is the best evidence for the novelty of wind as "the chief of the hundred diseases." The concept of empty winds belonged to a new vision of the world. To recognize time gone awry, even to conceive the idea, one must have already a precise prescription for time's proper course, exact expectations about what events should occur when. One must demand a cosmos ruled by rhythm.[60] This rhythm had a name: *bafeng sishi*, the eight winds and four seasons.

Sometime near the end of the Warring States period, writers began to speak of eight winds (*bafeng*) instead of four, and to call these eight by special names; in Qin and early Han times, the nomenclature was still in flux.[61] This innovation refined the traditional partition of space by introducing breezes from the northeast, southeast, southwest, and northwest between the four cardinal winds. More critically, it advanced an altered sense of time.

In Shang divination, the cardinal wind spirits served the capricious Emperor (*Di*). Oracle inscriptions ask: "Will Di send wind on this day?" "Should we sacrifice three dogs so that Di will order forth wind?" "Will wind blow from the east?" "Will wind blow from the west?" — evoking a world in which winds arose, twisted in new directions, and died, unpredictably, erratically, like the whims of a moody tyrant.

The Han-dynasty diviner Zhao Da inhabited a very different world. He scoffed at those who tracked winds outside, in harsh weather, for he reached his predictions in the comfort of his home.[62] Archaeological excavations in 1977 unearthed divining boards of the sort used by Zhao's school, shedding light on his condescension: Zhao's technique relied more on numerical calculations than direct observation.[63] It presumed a predictable system in wind's shifts.

The eightfold division of space anchored a division of the year into eight forty-five-day segments, each ruled by a particular wind. Beginning with the easterly breezes, which brought spring, winds made their way clockwise around the wind rose — from east to southeast, to south, and so on to northeast, and finally back to

254

east. In the course of the Han dynasty, *bafeng sishi* became a stock formula, affirming the inseparability of the eight winds and four seasons, of wind and time.

Han divining boards tied this circulation of winds to the migration of a deity, Taiyi, around "nine palaces" — the eight directions and the center. Winds blowing from the palace occupied by Taiyi were full winds; empty winds were those that blew from palaces where Taiyi was absent. This is why proper winds were synonymous with full winds, and why irregular evil winds were also termed empty.

As evident in the coincidence of terms, the medical theory of full and empty winds drew heavily on this theory of divination. The most systematic analysis of wind etiology in the *Neijing*, in fact, appears in a treatise explicitly named "The Nine Palaces and Eight Winds (*jiugong bafeng*)."[64] Wind's power thus continued to hint of divine presence, just as in archaic times, but there was now an insistence on calculable cadences, on regular rhythms dictating even the movements of deities.

As we observed in chapter 4, Chinese medicine assumed its classical form at just the time when China developed, for the first time, into a unified, universal empire. During the Qin and Han dynasties, as rulers came to claim authority over all under heaven, assertions of correspondence between microcosm and macrocosm served effectively to buttress the political status quo. Elaborated in Han Confucianism through such schemes as the yin and yang and the five phases, the eight winds and four seasons, the rhetoric of human and heavenly resonance prescribed and justified the social order as a mirror of the natural order.

The diviner's insistence on a latent regularity *to* time paralleled the elaboration of a politics regulated *by* time. To the *bafeng*, eight winds, corresponded the *bazheng*, eight modes of government. When the east wind blew, marking the onset of spring,

255

those imprisoned for minor crimes were to be released. When the wind then shifted to the southeast, messengers bearing gifts of silk cloth were to be sent to the regional lords.[65] For each wind there were special robes to be worn, foods to be eaten, fixed rituals to be performed.

Precepts of personal regimen, too, shaded imperceptibly into guidelines for statecraft. In spring, the *Suwen* advises, "the myriad things flourish, engendered by heaven and earth together. Going to sleep at nightfall one should get up early and stride leisurely in the garden. Letting one's hair down and putting oneself at ease, one should give rise to one's ambitions. Engender and do not kill. Give and do not take away. Reward and do not punish. That is what befits the spirit of spring."[66] Managing the self and managing society demanded like disciplines.

But the synchrony of human life with the rhythm of the winds and seasons wasn't just or mainly a matter of conscious choice. It accompanied a sense of cosmic belonging whose full force we struggle now to appreciate. Just as trees changed foliage and animals frolicked or hibernated, the human body too had its seasons. In spring, the liver gained ascendance, in summer the heart, in autumn the lungs, in winter the kidneys. If Greek anatomists advanced a science of articulated forms, here was a body articulated by time. Easterly winds arose in spring and brought diseases to the neck and the back of the head; southerly winds arose in summer and caused diseases in the chest; westerly winds arose in autumn and hurt the shoulders and upper back; northerly winds arose in winter and attacked the lower back and legs.[67]

These were palpable changes, manifest to the touch. Crucial to knowing the body was a grasp of its seasonal feel. As spring became summer, then gave way to autumn, and then winter, different *zang* waxed and waned, and the flowing *mo* rose to the surface or receded to the depths: "In the spring, the *mo* is floating, like fish playing in the waves. In the summer, the *mo* overflows the skin, and the myriad things know superabundance. In the autumn, the *mo* is below the skin, and the insects prepare to leave. In the winter, the *mo* is at the bones, the insects hibernate."[68]

The theory of winds was thus a theory of time. Not a cool and transparent geometrical time, a line without breadth or depth stretching into infinity, or even a repeating circle, but rather a real presence, perceptible change felt with the skin, smelled, seen, heard. It was the atmosphere that we sense in winter when walking down a country road we see people huddled around a crackling fire; or the feel of spring when we hear the splashing of fish in the creek, or see insects and animals emerging from the ground. It was a seasonal spirit that at once transformed the surrounding plants and animals and paced the cadences of inner life.

But this is just half the story.

There was a tension at the heart of Chinese medicine. At the same time that it celebrated the resonance of microcosm and macrocosm, it asserted the body's latent independence from wind. Despite the rootedness of human being in the world, despite the confluence of cosmic winds and personal spirit, the body remained separate from the world around it.

Modern accounts of Chinese medical thought have generally underplayed this ambivalence, ignoring the powerful pull toward isolation. Yet both the compulsion to preserve vital fullness and the fear of depletion and invasion — core themes, we discovered before, in Chinese appreciations of health and sickness — presupposed a sharp divide between outer gales and breezes and inner essential breaths. Independence from the volatility of winds defined the very possibility of security in life, the dream of autonomy.

Why should people ever fall sick? If the cycle of seasons ran steady and if all lives changed in unison with the seasonal spirit, sickness shouldn't even exist. Yet sickness is actually pervasive. Why? Often to blame were erratic, empty winds. At times, the seasons got out of kilter; at times, time itself went awry.

Reflected in the rise of wind as "the chief of the hundred diseases" was a new sensitivity to chaos. Exhortations to harmonize with cosmic change presupposed the predictable regularity of the eight winds and four seasons. But this same predictability also fostered a keener awareness of winds arriving too soon, too late, out of turn.

In this sense, the medical preoccupation with empty winds went hand-in-hand with the establishment of the theory of cosmic harmonies. Empty winds were winds that thwarted expectations, transgressed against cosmic propriety. They embodied contingency and chance, the obstinate halo of uncertainty that made all science mere approximation. Because they arose unexpectedly, spontaneously, irregularly, because they made harsh, abrupt shifts, winds became associated especially with the most dramatic, sudden afflictions — with strokes, epilepsy, madness. It was wind's protean volatility, its lack of regularity (*wuchang*), that made it "the origin of the hundred diseases."

Separating and protecting human beings from the wind's volatile whimsy were the skin and pores. It was the skin that wind, rain, and cold first attacked, and it was through the pores that they penetrated into the body.[69] When read together with skin complexion, the pores thus gave insight into inner powers. In a person with red complexion (the color associated with the heart) fine-grained pores signaled a small heart, while coarse pores indicated a large heart. In a person with white complexion (the color corresponding to the lungs) fine-grained pores bespoke small lungs, and coarse pores large lungs.[70]

Lingshu 47 observes more generally that when the body's protective breaths (*weiqi*) are harmonized, the sinews are flexible, the skin is pliant, and the pores closely knit (*zouli zhimi*).[71] Therefore, adds *Lingshu* 50, those with thin skin and flabby flesh succumb to untimely winds, those with thick skin and firm flesh do not.[72] The skin and pores at once manifested the strength within a person and gave protection from the dangers without. If one hoped to live long and free from sickness, it was vital that the blood and *qi* flow unobstructed, the five flavors be regulated, the bones straight, the sinews pliant, and, note well, the pores closely knit (*mi*).[73] When the flesh and pores are closed tight, then even great gales can inflict no harm.[74] One thus had to avoid winds after exertions, when sweat poured out and the pores were agape. So many sudden catastrophes struck in the form of winds rushing in through loose, unguarded pores.[75] Tight pores at once signified and assured vitality, demarcating and safeguarding self from surrounding chaos.

Today we speak but metaphorically of the "winds of change." The vigilance with which doctors monitored the skin and pores, however, reminds us that the discourse of winds once gave voice to an embodied experience of space and time, a physical feel for local airs, seasonal atmosphere, shifting moods, contingency. Personal breaths could harmonize with cosmic breath, and habitually the two might be reasonably in phase; but nothing could make all chance disappear. This was the ultimate truth of wind — that always, at any moment, it could abruptly turn and blow toward unknown horizons.

Embodiment and Change

Greek wind consciousness also evolved. But rather than gain in menace, as they did in China, winds in Greek medicine drifted instead toward the periphery of concerns.

After Hippocrates we find faint trace of the sense, so vivid in works like the *Sacred Disease* and *Airs, Waters, Places,* of wind's

259

ubiquitous presence. Neither Herophilus nor Erasistratus, as far as we can tell, tracked wind's shifts like the author of *Epidemics* 1; and in all of Galen's prolific production only one treatise — his commentary on the Hippocratic treatise *On Humors*, and within that only one chapter — discusses winds at any length.[76] Elsewhere, in over twenty thick volumes of Galen's collected works, we can glean only a handful of scattered, passing references.[77]

Arguments from silence are necessarily inconclusive, of course, but in this case there is also suggestive testimony of another sort. For doctors after Hippocrates didn't actually stop speaking of *pneuma*. They merely spoke of them in an altered sense. If they lingered less on cold northerly blasts and the warm breezes wafting up from the south, they developed more fine-grained analyses of breaths within the body, innate powers, soul.

This may be one reason why historians of medicine so rarely mention winds in their surveys. Historiography here reflects history: over the course of antiquity winds began already to recede significantly from medical consciousness.[78] Studies of *pneuma*, accordingly, concentrate almost exclusively on internal "wind," vital breath. Verbeke's classic, *L'Evolution de la doctrine du pneuma*, tells the tale of *pneuma*'s *spiritualization*, tracing how the material breath of physicians like Alcmaeon gradually evolved into the immaterial *spiritus* of Christianity.[79] He says nothing of *pneumata* as northerly and southerly breezes. Include the earlier history of *pneuma* as wind, though, and the process of dematerialization appears as part of a broader trajectory — a drift toward *internalization*. Instead of tracking the airs that shaped human life from without, doctors became increasingly captivated by the notion of breaths shaping and animating human beings from within. The Galenic body differed from the Hippocratic not just in its richer structural detail, that is, not just because of the new science of dissection, but also in an altered awareness of *pneuma*.

Is there a connection between these two — between the emergence of the anatomical eye and the shift in pneumatic intuitions?

Belief in ties between breath and being was hardly new. Aeschylus' warriors breathed *menos*, the *Sacred Disease* linked consciousness to the unobstructed flow of air. Possible consequences of blocked breath, adds the appendix to *Regimen in Acute Diseases*, include trembling, heaviness in the head, clouded vision.[80] Northerly and southerly winds shaped not only people's character and passing moods, but their visible form as well.

Yet we have seen that in classical drama and in the Hippocratic writings winds and breaths habitually blended into each other, without definite demarcations. By contrast, one of the distinctive features of Aristotle's theory of connate *pneuma* (*symphyton pneuma*) was that it posited an innate breath independent of seasonal or regional winds, an inner power, moreover, decisive for the body's form. The connate *pneuma* gave shape to the blood in the womb and molded and articulated the fetus — informing the body from within, as a fiery breath expanding outward rather than as winds carving up physiques from the outside. And once the inner structures were fully articulated, the connate *pneuma* then ensured their stability; by themselves, the four elements could neither create shapes nor preserve them.[81]

Greek doctors throughout antiquity, then, imagined *pneumata* affecting how people look, feel, and act. But whereas in Hippocratic works like *Airs, Waters, Places*, *Sacred Disease*, and *Epidemics* 1 and 3 *pneumata* were winds that provided, as it were, the *context* of human being, writers from Aristotle through Galen elaborated *pneuma* as inner *content*. To be sure, Galen's psychic *pneuma* had roots in the earlier pneumatism of Diogenes and the *Sacred Disease* and was fed by air drawn in from the outside; but once inside the body this air had to be substantially altered — become subtler, lighter — before it flowed through the brain and nerves and made possible thought, sensation, and movement. For Christians like Origen and Augustine, *spiritus* would constitute nothing less than a divine essence, a person's inner core.[82]

We tend now to take for granted that a doctor's training should begin with the study of inner structures and functions, with mastery of anatomy and physiology. But there was an era when the body represented something quite different from the entity that we imagine now — a discrete given, an independent and isolated object. Once upon a time, all reflection on what we call the body was inseparable from inquiry into places and directions, seasons and winds. Once upon a time, human being was being embedded in a world.

The decline of this awareness is a long and complex tale. The certainty of ties between heavenly and earthly bodies made astrological consultation integral to medieval medicine. An influential neo-Hippocratic tradition continued periodically up through the nineteenth century to dwell on the claims of climate and air.[83] Fully to trace the erosion of this meteorological consciousness, moreover, we would have to stalk many developments after antiquity — the Renaissance culture of dissection, the nineteenth-century clinical gaze, the contemporary reign of technology.

Nevertheless, the internalization of *pneuma* in antiquity represented a momentous turn — one that helped to place anatomical knowledge firmly at the core of medical knowledge.[84] For it redefined the nature of the body.

We must distinguish, the Hippocratic treatise *On Ancient Medicine* tells us, between illnesses due to "forces" and illnesses due to "forms": "By forces I mean those changes in the constitution of the humors which affect the working of the body; by forms I mean the organs of the body."[85] Thus runs the rendering of Chadwick and Mann. Littré similarly translates the last half: "J'appelle figures la conformation des organes qui sont dans le corps." However, the original Greek sentence doesn't actually speak of organs. It refers only to "those [things] that are in a human being" (*hosa enestin en toi anthrōpoi*).[86]

The Chadwick and Mann translation goes on to describe "organs that attract moisture," "solid and round organs," and "organs which are more spread out." Organs "which are spongy and of loose texture such as the spleen, the lungs, and the female breasts," we learn,

> easily absorb fluid from the nearby parts of the body and when they do so become hard and swollen. Such organs do not absorb fluid and then discharge it day after day as would a hollow organ containing fluid, but when they have absorbed fluid and all the spaces and interstices are filled up, they become hard and tense instead of soft and pliant. They neither digest the fluid nor discharge it, and this is the natural result of their anatomical construction.[87]

Now organ (*organon*) is a good Greek word, but it appears nowhere in *Ancient Medicine*. All the references to "organs" in this translation, as well as the tendentious phrase "anatomical construction," render another Greek word: *schēma*, form or shape. And shapes obviously are what this passage is about. From their shapes follow naturally and necessarily the properties of the various parts — their propensity to attract moisture or not, to retain fluids or to repel them.

The theory of a body constructed around organs matured only after Hippocrates, and when it matured the theory was emphatically not — and this is why terminology matters — a theory of processes that occur naturally, of themselves. It was a theory of *action*. Galen explains: "I call organ a part of the animal that is the cause of a complete action, as the eye is of vision, the tongue of speech, and the legs of walking; so too arteries, veins and nerves are both organs and parts of animals."[88]

Body parts may be distinguished in many ways — by their size or shape, their color, location, or texture. What made a part an *organ*, however, was its role in some activity, the enabling of acts like seeing, talking, walking. *Organa* were tools — the original meaning of the term — instruments with specific uses. And they presupposed a *user*.

Popular writings currently tend to tie the Western emphasis on dissection to a reductionist, mechanistic stance toward the body, and to contrast this mechanism with the alleged "organicism" of Chinese healing. But this view is historically indiscriminate. It forgets that the traditional anatomical perception of the body as an organization of organs required the presence of an active soul. "The usefulness of all the organs," Galen declares, "is related to the soul. For the body is the instrument of the soul, and consequently animals differ greatly in respect to their parts because their souls also differ. For some animals are brave and others timid, some are wild and others tame.... In every case the body is adapted to the character and faculties of the soul."[89]

Chapter 3 drew attention to intuitions of purposive action which framed Greek dissection. Crucial to seeing the body anatomically was seeing each part as a structure fashioned for some end. The concept of organs further tightens, now, the bonds between action and anatomy. For it suggests how active purpose not only steered the original formation of the body, but also animated its parts.

Soul and the organic body were linked from the beginnings of anatomy. Aristotle, who pioneered dissection as a way of knowing, also forged the theory of organism — the idea of the body as an implement. "Just as mind acts with some purpose in view," he urged, "so too does nature, and this purpose is its end. In living

264

creatures the soul supplies such a purpose . . . for all natural bodies are instruments of the soul."[90]

By the seventeenth century, of course, this view faced increasing challenges. Iatrophysicists began to analyze the body's workings in purely mechanical terms, and the Cartesian conception of mind as pure reflection — the retraction of the soul from the body — spurred the new concept of reflex, a bodily action occurring without the intervention of the soul. But belief in organs and the rule of inner breaths, the sense of a pneumatic soul, faded only gradually. In 1686, Daniel Duncan could still summarize: "The soul is a skilled organist, which forms its organs before playing them. It is a remarkable thing that in inanimate organs, the organist is different from the air that he causes to flow, whereas in animate organs the organist and the air that causes them to play are one and the same thing, by which I mean that the soul is extremely similar to the air or to breath."[91]

Chinese conceptions of the body's interior centered around the five *zang* and six *fu*. The five *zang* were the liver, heart, spleen, lungs, and kidneys; the six *fu* included the gall bladder, small intestines, stomach, large intestines, and bladder.[92] Reading casually, we might say: here is a list of organs.

A modern Chinese textbook cautions, though, that we "cannot simply impose Western medicine's conception of the internal organs" to the concepts of *zang* and *fu*; and Nathan Sivin adds, "[W]hat we learn about the Chinese conception is not anatomical but physiological and pathological . . . not what the viscera are but what they do in health and sickness."[93] The observation is accurate. Discussions of the *zang* and *fu* in the *Neijing* typically have to do less with discrete structures seen in dissection than with configurations of sympathetic powers. "Gall bladder disease" thus could refer as easily to disorders like dizziness or ringing in the ears as to an affliction in the gall bladder itself. When scholars insist that Chinese viscera differ from Western organs, this is what they usually mean: the *zang* and *fu* weren't anatomically conceived.

They also differed from the organs of Greek medicine in another, subtler way. The *zang* and the *fu* weren't tools of some controlling source, weren't implements of the soul. Literally, *zang* and *fu* both referred to repositories, and therein lay their principal role in the body. They both stored *qi*, vital breath.

The *fu* were hollow depots, like the stomach, intestines, and bladder, which temporarily housed the coarser, turbid essences, then passed them on, while *zang* named the solid viscera that "cache (*zang*) the refined *qi* and don't let it to escape."[94] The *zang* were more vital, both because they stored the purer essences and because they *retained* them; and among the *zang*, the kidneys were most vital, because they cached the most refined *qi*. The hierarchy structuring the Chinese body was defined not by the logic of ruler and ruled, but by the imperatives of storage and retention.

Modern expositions of Chinese medicine have habitually stressed theories like the yin, the yang, and the five phases — universalizing schemes that embed a microcosmic body in the macrocosmic order. Ilza Veith, the first scholar to attempt an extensive translation of the *Huangdi neijing*, thus explained:

> The earliest Chinese were awed by the immutable course of nature which they called Tao, the Way.... The dual force through which Tao acts was yin and yang.... Both yin and yang were held to be conveyed through the body by means of twelve hypothetical main channels, or Ching Lo, which correspond to the twelve months of the year.... [In] man, health resulted from a balance of yin and yang, and all diseases were thought to be due to an imbalance of these forces.[95]

266

Manfred Porkert's widely cited monograph, *The Theoretical Foundations of Chinese Medicine*, likewise bears the telling subtitle "Systems of Correspondence," and the opening three chapters discuss first the yin and yang and the five phases, second the rhythms of cosmic change, and third the reflection of macrocosmic order in the microcosm of the body.

No one could deny, of course, that familiarity with the yin and the yang and the five phases is indispensable for understanding Chinese medical writings. But it is also important to recognize that these writings also highlight, and elaborate in detail, the impact of factors that present-day accounts acknowledge with only brief, perfunctory nods. I mean the menace of heat and cold, humidity, dryness, and especially wind. Alongside the rhetoric of cosmic harmonies, we find an opposing ideal of being, one that envisioned the body as a self-contained reality, ruled by its own inner logic.

Mirrored in this ambivalence was the ambiguity of wind. Han dynasty cosmology banished unruly chaos by decree, declaring the rule of regularity, and aggressively framing change within the rhythms of the yin and the yang, the five phases, the eight winds and four seasons. Yet the very effort to impose order crystallized awareness of unpredictable chance, the persisting menace of empty winds.

If the authoritarian vision of universal order spoke of harmony and balance and promoted the seamless unity of self and the world, wariness of chaos inspired an opposing impulse toward timeless isolation, the dream of an autonomous self, impervious to wind's whimsy. The melding of microcosm and macrocosm thus represented but one facet of Chinese aspirations for the body. Doctors insisted just as adamantly on the separateness of an inside from an outside, the latent independence of the self from the world. Hence the attention, for example, devoted to what separated the two. Tight, closely knit pores guarded the self against incursions from without.

Real security, however, lay in inner fullness. To the extent that the *zang* storehouses kept vital breaths secure within the body, a person could deflect the perils of chaotic change. Empty winds could inflict no harm, for the fullness within left them no room to enter. The *Lingshu* asseverated: it is only when an untimely wind encounters depletion within the body that it can possess the body.[96] No principle was more basic to Chinese thinking about sickness.

For deflecting outer chaos wasn't the sole advantage. Fullness worked, too, against the steadier erosions of age. By carefully hoarding vitality, by not allowing desire to drain the body of life, a person could defer the approach of decline and death, delay the passing of the years. This is why Chinese texts of regimen so often speak of freedom from sickness together, in the same breath, with long life — why we can see old men modeling the routines of yogic discipline (figure 26). Health was virtually synonymous with longevity, immunity to change.[97]

From outer breezes, then, to inner breaths; from the unpredictable turns of fortune's winds to change paced internally, by autonomous selves. Such broad shifts marked conceptions of the body in both Greek and Chinese thinking. But autonomy in the two traditions was defined by two different approaches to time. The fullness of yogic figures in China (figures 22 and 23) portrayed selves preserving their integrity by resisting the depleting outflow of life, the loss of vital energies and of time. Whereas the autonomy of the muscleman lay in the capacity for genuine action, for change due neither to nature nor chance, but dependent solely on the will.

"As for what is known as the art of medicine," asserts Plato's *Epinomis*, "it also is, of course, a form of defense against the ravages committed on the living organism by the seasons with their untimely cold and heat and the like." Doctors are our defenders.

> But none of their devices can bestow reputation for the truest wisdom; they are at sea on an ocean of fanciful conjecture, without reduction to rule. We may also give the name of defender to sea captains and their crews, but I would have no one encourage our hopes by the proclamation that any of them is wise. None of them can know of the fury or kindness of the winds, and that is the knowledge coveted by every navigator.[98]

Just as sea captains defend ships against shifting winds, so it is the doctor's task to protect the body against unseasonal hot and cold.

The analogy is shrewdly calculated. In the *Statesman*, Plato again invokes seamanship and medicine together, equating the former with studies of nautical practice, and the latter with inquiry into "winds and temperatures."[99] For this contemporary of Hippocrates, then, the doctor's first concern was with the weather — that is, with inscrutable winds. This dependence on "the fury or kindness of the winds," common to doctors and sea captains alike, made both their arts fatally contingent. It prevented both medicine and navigation from becoming true sciences. For winds could never be truly known.

Plato's resignation to medicine's uncertainty later gave way to the Galenic conception of medicine as an axiomatic edifice patterned on geometrical method, a science based on fixed truths, rather than the art of handling chance.[100] For Galen, the doctor's apprenticeship no longer began with the study of winds — capricious influences molding human beings from the outside — but had to be grounded instead on the craftsmanlike logic organizing life from within. Where *Airs, Waters, Places* surveyed the sculpting of physiques by local airs, the anatomical forms admired by the dissector reflected the purposeful articulation of matter by innate breath.[101] Parts ceased to be mere shapes, *schēma*, and became organs, implements of the soul; and muscles, in particular, were born as the organs of voluntary motion, actions determined by the self. Where once *pneuma* served luck, in the flexing of muscles it expressed decisive will.

Hidden by their physical transparency and by centuries of oblivion, winds are invisible in the pictures that introduced this book. Yet to overlook their latent presence in figures 1 and 2 would be to miss a crucial part of what these illustrations mean. For the capaciousness of one body and the muscularity of the other portrayed, among other things, differing answers to a problem once posed most forcefully by wind, namely, how to imagine human being in a world of ceaseless change.

Epilogue

What separates the living from the dead?

Life's presence is manifest to the senses, yet ever eludes the reach of our comprehension. We plainly see the metamorphoses of vitality in someone running, stopping, looking back, turning pale; we can hear the supple force of life in the sharpness of precise diction, and in the soft insinuations of tone; we can even grasp vital power with our fingers, here at the wrist, feel it pulsating or flowing. But in the end, the mystery persists. Say that a living person possesses a soul, or spirit, or vital breath, and we have only invented names for ignorance.

It is ultimately into this mystery that we peer when we survey the disagreements among past accounts of the body. For if by the body we mean something directly accessible to sight and to touch, then, in the history of medicine, the body was no more the real object of knowledge than individual printed letters are the final object of reading. Just as letters interest the reader mainly as sensible bearers of insensible meaning, so in taking the pulse or feeling the *mo*, in dissecting muscles or scrutinizing color, doctors strove above all to comprehend what the body *expressed*. They sought to know the invisible, inaudible, intangible truth of living beings through bodily expressions that could be seen, and heard, and touched — to work back from manifest signs to their secret vital source.

271

The truth, however, is that there is no unique road back and there are no fixed and unmistakable signs. A vast chasm gapes between the inescapably limited scope of human awareness in any given era at any given place and the unknowable boundless plenitude of life's manifestations. Changes and features that speak eloquently to experts in one culture can thus seem mute and insignificant, and pass unnoticed, in another. Greek pulse takers ignored the local variations that their counterparts in China found so richly telling; Chinese doctors saw nothing of muscular anatomy. This is how conceptions of the body diverge — not just in the meanings that each ascribes to bodily signs, but more fundamentally in the changes and features that each recognizes *as* signs. Differences in the history of medical knowledge turn as much around what and how people perceive and feel (at once apprehending the body as an object, and experiencing it as embodied beings) as around what they think.

I have presented concrete illustrations of such differences in ancient Greek and Chinese medicine, and identified some of the factors that shaped them. I have proposed parallels between ways of touching and seeing on the one hand, and on the other, and ways of speaking and listening; I have stressed the inseparability of perceptions of the body and conceptions of personhood; and I have highlighted the interplay between the sense of embodied self and the experience of space and time. Throughout it all, however, I have also sought to convey a more general, and yet more intimate lesson. I have tried to suggest how comparative inquiry into the history of the body invites us, and indeed compels us, ceaselessly to reassess our own habits of perceiving and feeling, and to imagine alternative possibilities of being — to experience the world afresh. Such is the great challenge of charting the geography of medical understanding. And also its alluring promise.

Bibliographical Note

Unless otherwise specified, the volumes and page numbers of citations from the Hippocratic corpus and the writings of Galen refer, respectively, to the editions of Littré (abbrev. as L.) and Kühn (abbrev. as K.):

Emile Littré, ed., *Oeuvres complètes d'Hippocrate*, 10 vols. (Amsterdam: Adolf M. Hakkert, 1962; reprint of Paris, 1851 edition).

K. G. Kühn, ed., *Galenus; opera omnia*, 22 vols. (Hildesheim: G. Olms, 1964–65).

References to the *Suwen* and *Lingshu* are keyed to the *Huangdi neijing zhangju suoyin* (Taipei: Qiyen Shuju, 1987) and cite the standard treatise number followed by the page number in this edition. Thus Suwen 17/50 means *Suwen* treatise 17, p. 50.

YBQS is an abbreviation for the *Yibu quanshu* (Taipei: Wenyi Yinshuguan, 1977). The page numbers refer to vol. 3 of this collection.

Page references for the works below cite the following editions:

Guoyu = *Guoyu. Zhanguoce* (Changsha: Yuelu Shushe, 1988).

Hanfeizi (Taipei: Zhonghua Shuju, 1982).

Hanshu, 5 vols. (Taipei: Dingwen Shuju, 1981).

Liezi (Beijing: Wenxue Guji Kanxingshe, 1956).

Liji = *Liji zhengyi*, 2 vols. (Shanghai: Guji Chubanshe, 1990).

Lunheng = Huang Hui, ed., *Lunheng jiaoshi*, 2 vols. (Taipei: Shang-wu Yinshuguan, n.d.).

Shanghanlun (Taipei: Zhonghua Shuju, 1987).

Shiji, 6 vols. (Hong Kong: Zhonghua Shuju, 1969).

Shujing = *Shangshu zhengyi* (Taipei: Zhonghua Shuju, 1979).

Zhanguoce = *Zhanguoce jizhu huikao*, 3 vols. (Jiangsu Guji Chu-banshe, 1985).

Zuozhuan = *Chunqiu zuozhuan jinzhu jinshi*, 3 vols. (Taipei: Shang-wu Yinshuguan, 1987).

Notes

PREFACE

1. Paul Valéry, "Aesthetics," in his *Collected Works in English* (Princeton, NJ: Princeton University Press, 1964), vol. 13.

CHAPTER ONE: GRASPING THE LANGUAGE OF LIFE

1. John Donne, *Devotions upon Emergent Occasions* (London: Simkin, Marshall, Hamilton, Kent Co., n.d.; originally published 1624), Meditation 1, 9–10.

2. *Plutarch's Lives*, trans. J. Langhorne and W. Langhorne, 8 vols., (London: J. Richardson and Co., 1821), vol. 7, 240.

3. Sima Qian, *Shiji*, chap. 105, 2785–2820, esp. 2798–99, 2801, 2804–5, 2807.

4. Cao Xueqin, *The Story of the Stone*, trans. David Hawkes (New York: Penguin, 1973), vol. 1, 224–25.

5. Pierre Huard and C. Wong, "Bio-bibliographie de la médecine chinoise," *Bulletin de la Société des Etudes Indochinoises* 31 (1956): 200.

6. Quoted in Emmet Field Horine, "An Epitome of Ancient Pulse Lore," *Bulletin of the History of Medicine* 10 (1941): 227.

7. Benjamin Rush, "On the Pulse," *Medical and Surgical Reporter* (Philadelphia) 45 (1881): 311.

8. R. Vance, "The Doctrine of the Pulse: An Analysis of Its Character and Summary of Its Indications," *Cincinnati Lancet and Observer* 26 (1878): 360.

9. Julius Rucco, *Introduction to the Science of the Pulse* (London, 1827), ii.

10. Lu Gwei-djen and Joseph Needham, *Celestial Lancets: A History and Rationale of Acupuncture and Moxa* (Cambridge: Cambridge University Press, 1980), 37.

11. Jean Jacques Menuret de Chambaud, "Pouls," in *Encyclopédie, ou dictionnaire raisonné des sciences, des arts et des métiers* (Facsimile of edition of 1751–80) (Stattgart-Bad Cannstatt: Friedrich Frommann Verlag, 1966), vol. 13, 222.

12. Cited in Boleslaw Szczesniak, "John Floyer and Chinese Medicine," *Osiris* 11 (1954): 154–55.

13. Menuret de Chambaud, "Pouls," 222.

14. John Floyer, *The Physician's Pulse Watch* (London: Samuel Smith and Benjamin Walford, 1707), 354–55.

15. Floyer, *Physician's Pulse Watch*, 228. The passage continues: "Samedo the Portuguese commends them for their skill, and says they never ask their patients any questions, they feel the pulse in both hands laid on a pillow; and they observe their motions a great while, and afterwards tell what the patient aileth; and he farther saith, that the good and learned physicians seldom fail; and he also observes that . . . by the pulse they can tell all the alterations in diseases."

16. Charles Ozanam, *La Circulation et le pouls: Histoire, physiologie, sémiotique, indications thérapeutiques* (Paris: Librairie J.B. Baillière et Fils, 1886), 84.

17. On the vagaries of Chinese pulse diagnosis in Europe, the best account remains Mirko Grmek, "Les Reflets de la sphygmologie chinoise dans la médecine occidentale," *Biologie médicale* 51 (1962). See also Rolf Winau, "Chinesische Pulsdiagnostik in 17. Jahrhundert in Europa," in *Medizinische Diagnostik in Geschichte und Gegenwart*, eds. Christa Habrich et al. (Munich: Werner Fritsch, 1978), 61–70.

18. For a review of the debate surrounding the question of which, if any, of the works in the Hippocratic corpus are the genuine works of Hippocrates, see G.E.R. Lloyd, "The Hippocratic Question," *Classical Quarterly* 25 (1975): 171–92. On the formation of the Hippocratic corpus and the image of Hippocrates over the ages, see Wesley Smith, *The Hippocratic Tradition* (Ithaca, NY: Cornell University Press, 1979).

An excellent starting point for orienting oneself among the editions of Galen's works is Vivian Nutton's *Karl Gottlob Kühn and his Edition of the Works of Galen: A Bibliography* (Oxford: Oxford Microform Publications, 1976). Early Latin collections of Galen's work are reviewed by Loren C. MacKinney in *Isis* 41 (1950): 199–201. John Scarborough critically reviews the traditions concerning Galen's life and works in "The Galenic Question," *Sudhoffs Archiv* 65 (1981): 1–31.

19. Charles Daremberg and Charles Emile Ruelle, eds., *Oeuvres de Rufus d'Ephèse* (Amsterdam: Adolf M. Hakkert, 1963; reprint of the 1879 Paris edition), 219.

20. Galen mentions him several times in connection with this treatise, *On Palpitations*, but he shows himself uncertain both about which Aegimius it is a question of, and about whether in fact Aegimius was the author of this work. (See *Peri diaphoras sphygmōn* 1.2 (K.8.498); *ibid.*, 4.2 (K.8.716); *ibid.* 4.11 (K.8.751–52). See also Daremberg's remarks in his notes to this opening passage (Daremberg and Ruelle, 625–26).

21. *Peri diaphoras sphygmōn* 1.2 (K.8.498).

22. Daremberg and Ruelle, 615–18; C.R.S. Harris, *The Heart and the Vascular System in Ancient Greek Medicine* (Oxford: Clarendon Press, 1973), 185.

23. Galen's analysis bears mention here. The ancient physicians, according to him, applied the term *sphyzein* only to inflammations and to movements induced by inflammation, and never to the healthy parts of the body. He speculates that *sphygmos* referred not to all the movements of the arteries, but only to those great and violent movements perceptible to the patient himself (*Peri diaphoras sphygmōn* 4.2 [K.8.716]). The ancients here most likely do not include Hippocrates, for there are several passages in the Corpus which clearly point to pulsation as sensed by the physician rather than subjectively sensed by the patient. Moreover, Galen clearly distinguishes Hippocrates from these ancients on two occasions (*Quod animi mores corporis temperamenta sequantur* 8 [K.4.804], *Hippocratis de humoribus liber et Galeni in eum commentarii* 1.24 [K.16.203]).

24. *Peri agmōn* 25 (L.3.500); *Peri helkōn* 1 (L.6.400); *Epidēmiōn* 4.20 (L.5.158). It is perhaps an extension of this notion of feverishness that in

Epidēmiōn 2 a patient whose vessel (*phleps*) pulsates at the elbow is diagnosed as either liable to madness or quick-tempered (*Epidēmiōn* 2.5 [L.5.131]).

25. *Epidēmiōn* 2.6 (L.5.134).

26. The idea of the perpetual movement of the heart and blood vessels is not totally absent, however. A passage from *Peri sarkōn* 6 (L.8.592) reads, "The heart and the hollow vessels (*koilai phlebes*) always move," and *Peri topōn tōn kata anthrōpon* 3 (L.6.280) notes that in the temples are vessels that always pulse (*sphyzousin*). But such passages are rare. The author of *Peri physōn* 8 (L.6.104), moreover, treats this movement in the temples as pathological. See also *Peri diaphoras sphygmōn* 4.2 (K.8.716); 4.3 (K.8.723–4); Daremberg and Ruelle, 220–21.

27. Noteworthy in this regard is the absence of any reference to the pulse in passages (e.g., *Epidēmiōn* 1.23, *Peri technēs* 13) detailing the diagnostic signs to which a doctor should pay attention.

28. *Gynaikeōn* 2.120 (L.8.262); *Epidēmiōn* 4.23 (L.5.164).

29. *Peri nousōn* 2.4, 12, 16 (L.7.10, 22, 30).

30. *Kōakai prognōsies* 2.15 (L.5.648), 2.19 (L.5.660); *Epidēmiōn* 5.11 (L.5.210).

31. There are nonetheless some interesting tendencies in usage. For example, *palmos* is the preferred term for naming the paranormal palpitations of the heart or the body as a whole (*Humors* 9 [L.5.490], *Prorrhētikos* 30 [L.5.518], *Kōakai prognōsies* 2.18 [L.5.656]), while *sphyzein* is the verb usually associated with the pulsation in the temples (*Peri diaitēs okseōn (Notha)* 8 [L.2.427]; *Epidēmiōn* 7.3 and 25 [L.5.368, 370, 394]).

32. See Fritz Steckerl, *The Fragments of Praxagoras of Cos and His School* (Leiden: E.J. Brill, 1958).

33. *Synopsis* 2 (Daremberg and Ruelle, 220); Galen, *Peri tromou kai palmou kai spasmou kai rigous* 1 (K.2.584).

34. *Peri palmōn*, edited by Hermann Diels in *Abhandlungen der Preussischen Akademie der Wissenschaften, Philologie-historische Klasse* 4 (1907). On palmo-mantics, see "Palmoskopia" in *Paulys Real-Encyclopädie de classischen Alterumwissenschaft* (Waldsee: Alfred Druckenmüller, 1949), "Palatinus bis Parantellonta," 261–62.

35. *Peri diaphoras sphygmōn* 4.2 (K.8.716); 4.3 (K.8.723–24). Also Daremberg and Ruelle, 220–21.

36. *On Respiration* 480a.

37. *On Respiration* 479b.

38. Daremberg and Ruelle, 219–20.

39. *Peri hiērēs nosou* 6; *Peri physios anthrōpou* 11. Also see Aristotle, *History of Animals* 3.2, 511b.

40. On Herophilus, see esp. Heinrich von Staden, *Herophilus: The Art of Medicine in Early Alexandria* (Cambridge: Cambridge University Press, 1989). Earlier studies include J.F. Dobson, "Herophilus of Alexandria," *Proceedings of the Royal Society of Medicine* 18 (1925), 19ff; Peter Fraser, *Ptolemaic Alexandria* (Oxford: Clarendon Press, 1984) vol. 1, 348–64; F. Kudlien, "Herophilos und der Beginn der medizinischen Skepsis," in H. Flashar, *Antike Medizin* (Darmstadt: Wissenschaftliches Buches, 1971), 280–95.

41. Werner Jaeger, *Hermes* 48 and 62. Praxagoras's priority, however, is not beyond question. See Steckerl, *Praxagoras of Cos*, 17 n. 1.

42. Steckerl, *Praxagoras*, 18.

43. Daremberg and Ruelle, 220; also *Peri tromou* 1 (K.7.584) and 5 (K.7.598).

44. *Peri diaphoras sphygmōn* 4.3 (K.8.723).

45. Daremberg and Ruelle, 221; also *Peri diaphoras sphygmōn* 4.2 (K.8.724).

46. Rufus, *Synopsis* 2 (trans. von Staden, *Herophilus*, 327).

47. *Peri diaphoras sphygmōn* 4.6 (K.8.732).

48. *Peri diaphoras sphygmōn* 4.10 (K.8.743); also Hermann Schöne, "Markellinos' Pulslehre," *Festschrift zur 49 Versammlung deutscher Philologen und Schulmänner* (Basel, 1907), 457.

49. *Peri diaphoras sphygmōn* 4.7 (K.8.734).

50. *Peri diagnōseōs sphygmōn* 1.2 (K.8.776–77); also *Peri diaphoras sphygmōn* 4.5 (K.8.729).

51. *Peri diaphoras sphygmōn* 4.4–5 (K.8.725–27).

52. *Peri diaphoras sphygmōn* 4.4–5 (K.8.726–32).

53. *Peri diaphoras sphygmōn* 4.2 (K.8.706).

54. *Peri diaphoras sphygmōn* 4.2 (K.8.710). This observation about the visi-

bility of arterial motion in thin individuals was not original to Galen and was already pointed out by Archigenes (*Peri diagnōseōs sphygmōn* 1.2 [K.8.779]).

55. *Peri diagnōseōs sphygmōn* 1.2 (K.8.786–87); Harris, *Heart and Vascular System*, 255.

56. Galen, *Horoi iatrikoi* 205 and 206 (K.19.402–3).

57. *Peri diagnōseōs sphygmōn* 1.1 (K.8.789). On the similarity between Galen's description of his haptic enlightenment and Plato's characterization of the philosopher's apprehension of the Good, see Karl Deichgräber, "Galen als Erforscher des menschlichen pulses," *Sitzungberichtge der deutschen Akademie der Wissenschaften zu Berlin; Klasse für Sprachen, Literatur und Kunst* (1956), 22–23.

58. *Peri diagnōseōs sphygmōn* 1.1 (K.8.770).

59. *Peri diagnōseōs sphygmōn* 1.3 (K.8.500).

60. *Peri diagnōseōs sphygmōn* 3.2 (K.8.895).

61. Floyer, *Physician's Pulse Watch*, 355.

62. Johann Ludwig Formey, *Versuch einer Wurdigung des Pulses* (Berlin: Rucker, 1823), 4–5.

63. Cited in Quan Hansheng, "Qingmo xiyang yixue chuanru shi guoren suo chi de taidu," *Shihuo* 3.12 (1936): 50.

64. Cited in Quan, "Qingmo," 53.

65. Assembling a mix of texts from diverse medical traditions, it was probably first compiled during the Han dynasty (221 B.C.E.–220 C.E.). However, this original text no longer survives, and the organization and some of the contents of the present *Neijing* are the product of later recensions. In addition to the *Suwen* and *Lingshu*, two other works, the *Jiayijing* and the *Taisu*, preserve the text of the original *Neijing*.

The complex history of the *Neijing*'s composition and transmission is the subject of ongoing research. The best introduction in English may be David Keegan, "The Forms of a Tradition: The Structure and History of the *Huang-ti nei-ching*," (Ph.D. diss., University of California, Berkeley, 1986) and Yamada Keiji, "The Formation of the Huang-ti Nei-ching," *Acta Asiatica* 36 (1979): 67–89. The latter first appeared in Japanese as "Kōtei daikei no seiritsu," *Shisō* 662 (1979): 94–108, and must be supplemented with Yamada Keiji, "Kyūkyū happū setsu to Shōshiha no tachiba," *Tōhō gakuhō* 52 (1980): 199–242. For Yamada's most recent interpretation of the geneaology of the *Neijing*, see his *Chūgoku igaku no shisōteki fūdo* (Tokyo: Asashio Shuppan, 1995).

66. On the evolution of diagnostic palpation in China, see Maruyama Masao, *Shinkyū igaku to koten no kenkyū*, pt. 4: "Myakushin no kenkyū" (Tokyo: Sōgensha, 1977), 191–236; Fujiki Toshirō, "Somon, Reisū, Nangyō ni okeru shakusun shinpō no hensen," in his *Shinkyū igaku genryū kō* (Tokyo: Sekibundō, 1979), 114–24; Liao Yuqun, "Suwen yu Lingshu zhong de mofa," in Yamada Keiji and Tanaka Tan, eds., *Chūgoku kodai kagakushi ron (zokuhen)* (Kyoto: Kyoto Daigaku Jimbun Kagaku Kenkyūjo, 1991), 493–511; Ren Yingqiu, *Zhongyi moxue shi jiang* (Hong Kong: Taiping Shuju, 1962). Paul Unschuld's translation of the *Nan-ching* (Berkeley: University of California Press, 1986) offers an English rendering of an important primary source and its commentaries. For introductory Western-language accounts of Chinese pulsetaking, see Shang Ch'i-tung, "L'Histoire du développement de l'art de prendre le pouls," *Chinese Journal of History of Medicine* 7 (1955): 95–99; P. Huard and M. Durand, "Lan-ōng et la médecine sino-viêtnamienne," *Bulletin de la Société Indochinoise* 28 (1953); K. Chimin Wong, "The Pulse Lore of Cathay," *China Medical Journal* 42 (1948): 884–97; and Mirko Grmek, "Les Reflets de la sphygmologie chinoise."

67. *Lingshu* 9/293–94; also *Suwen* 9/33.

68. *Suwen* 20/64–65.

69. *Suwen* 17/53.

70. However, some doctors identified them instead with the radial (outer) and ulnar (inner) halves of the pulse. See, e.g., Chu Yong, *Quyi shuo*, "Bian mo" (*YBQS*, 2107).

71. *Myakui bensei* (Kyoto, 1721).

72. Li Gao, *Shishu*, "Sanbu suozhu zangfu binglun" (*YBQS*, 2124).

73. *Peri tōn sphygmōn tois eisagomenois* 1 (K.8.454).

74. Most commentators have identified "outer" and "inner" with the superficial (*fu*) and sunken (*chen*) positions. On the uniformity of pulsation at all sites, see Galen, *De pulsuum dignotione* 2.3 (K.8.862–63). Medieval illustrations of pulse taking, however, sometimes depict the doctor examining the pulse at

the upper arm as well (figure 8). I have as yet been unable to determine the significance of this technique.

In the eighteenth century, the prestige and influence of Chinese ideas led some doctors to look more seriously at the local variability of pulse qualities. See, e.g., Menuret de Chambaud, "Pouls," 208–10. The unique earlier example that I have found, of using different finger positions to diagnose different organs is Mercurius, *De pulsibus* (J.L. Ideler, *Physici et medici graeci minores*, vol. 2 [Berlin, 1842], 254–55).

75. Zuozhuan Duke Xi year 15. Interestingly, the earliest representations of blood vessels in Greek sculpture also are found in reliefs of horses. Indeed, prior to their depiction in humans, blood vessels are apparently shown *only* in horses. See Guy P.R. Métraux, *Sculptors and Physicians in Fifth-Century Athens* (Montreal: McGill-Queen's University Press, 1995), 26.

76. On these texts and the Mawangdui materials more generally, see Ma Jixing, *Mawangdui gu ishu kaoshi* (Changsha: Hunan Kexue Jishu Chubanshe, 1992); Zhou Yimo, *Mawangdui yixue wenhua* (Shanghai: Wenhui Chubanshe, 1994). For text, commentary, and Japanese translation of these texts, see Yamada Keiji, ed., *Shin hatsugen Chūgoku kagakushi shiryō no kenkyū. Shakuchū hen* (Kyoto: Kyoto Daigaku Jimbun Kagaku Kenkyūjo, 1985), 87–125. Akabori Akira, "*In'yō jūichi kyūkyō* no kenkyū," *Tōhō gakuhō* 53 (1981): 299–339, focuses particularly on the *Yinyang shiyimo jiujing*. The interpretation of these texts on the *mo* must now be supplemented with the more complete versions of some texts found in the Zhangjiashan tombs: Gao Dalun, ed., *Zhangjiashan hanjian "Moshu" jiaoshi* (Chengdu: Chengdu Chubanshe, 1992).

77. Yamada, *Shakuchū hen*, 87.

78. Ma, *Mawangdui gu ishu kaoshi*, 87–104, and Ma Jixing, *Mawangdui hanmu yanjiu* (Changsha: Hunan Renmin Chubanshe, 1981); Zhou, *Mawangdui*, 15–22; 27–35. Yamada Keiji, "Shinkyū to tōeki no kigen. Kodai Chūgoku igaku keisei no futatsu no isō," in Yamada Keiji, ed., *Shin hatsugen Chūgoku kagakushi shiryō no kenkyū. Ronkō hen.* (Kyoto: Kyoto Daigaku Jimbun Kagaku Kenkyūjo, 1985), 3–122.

79. He Zhiguo, "Xihan renti jingmo qidiao kao," *Daziran tansuo* 14.3 (1993):

116–21; Liang Fangrong et al., "Cong Xihan renti jingmo qidiao kan zaoqi jing-luo xueshuo," *Zhongguo zhenjiu* (1996), no. 4: 49–52; Ma Jixing, "Shuang-baoshan Hanmu chutu de zhenjiu jingmo qimu renxing," *Wenwu* (1996), no.4: 55–65.

80. Zhou Yimo, *Mawangdui*, 18–21, presents a well-reasoned review of this debate about points and conduits.

81. Yamada Keiji, "Shinkyū to tōeki no kigen. Kodai Chūgoku igaku keisei no futatsu no isō," in Yamada Keiji, ed., *Shin hatsugen Chūgoku kagakushi shiryō no kenkyū. Ronkō hen.* (Kyoto: Kyoto Daigaku Jimbun Kagaku Kenkyūjo, 1985), 3–122.

82. Lu and Needham, *Celestial Lancets*, 25.

83. *Lingshu* 4/278; Zhang Zhongjing, *Shanghanlun* (Taipei: Zhonghua Shuju, 1987), juan 1 "Bian mo fa" and "Ping mo fa." For a discussion, see Maruyama, *Shinkyū igaku*, 194–96 and 200–208.

84. All the *cunkou* sites, interestingly, belonged to the lungs. And perhaps not by coincidence: to the extent that Chinese texts supposed a force driving the flow of blood, they pointed to the lungs and to breath rather than to the heart. The Song-dynasty physician Cui Zixu thus explained: "*Mo* does not move itself. It arrives by following the breath (*qi*). Breath moves and *mo* responds.... Breath is like the bellows; blood is like the swelling waves" (*Siyen juyao*, YBQS 2102 and 2216).

See also Tao Jiucheng: "*Mo* is blood. But *mo* does not move itself. It is really breath which makes it move"(*Zhuogenglu*, YBQS 2122).

85. Li Gao, *Neiwaishang bianhuo lun*, "Bian mo," in *Jin-Yuan si da yixuejia mingzhu jicheng* (Beijing: Zhongguo Zhongyiyao Chubanshe, 1995), 395.

86. Li Zhongzi, *Yizong bidu* (Sanyutang edition, 1774), "Shen wei xiantian ben, pi wei houtian ben lun," juan 2, 6a.

87. *Lingshu* 30/357.

88. *Suwen* 17/50.

89. Gao Dalun, ed., *Zhangjiashan*, 104; Zhou, *Mawangdui*, 24.

90. *Suwen* 5/23.

91. *Suwen* 10/36. *Nanjing* 4.

92. *Suwen* 18/54.

93. *Lingshu* 38/277.

94. *Suwen* 18/55.

95. *Suwen* 17/53.

96. Wang Shuhe, *Mojing* (Hong Kong: Taiping Shuju, 1961), 2.

97. *Mojing*, 3.

98. *Mojue*, "Bali mo" (YBQS 2079).

99. See the analysis of this character in Tōdō Akiyasu, ed., *Kanwa daijiten* (Tokyo: Gakushū Kenkyūsha, 1978), 1062. A dictionary of the latter Han dynasty, the *Shiming*, glosses the right part of the character as "the crooked flow of water."

100. A later dictionary, the *Tongshi* thus glosses *mo* as "the branching flow of blood and *qi* to the four limbs" (Tao Jiucheng, *Zhuogenglu*: YBQS 2122). *Suwen* 3/14: "When the *yin* is overwhelmed by the *yang* the *mo* flows superficially, rapidly, and wildly."

101. *Guanzi*, chap. 39: "Shuidi," juan 14, 1a.

102. *Lingshu* 12/312. Similarly in the *Taisu* (treatise 5) we find, "The twelve *jingmo* correspond in the outside world to the twelve rivers, and inside the body to the five viscera and six hollow organs;" and again, "In the human body there are also four seas and twelve rivers, and these rivers all flow into the seas." See Unno Kazutaka, "The Geographical Thought of the Chinese People: With Special Reference to Ideas of Terrestial Features," *Memoirs of the Tōyō Bunko* 41 (1983): 90–95.

103. *Lunheng,* juan 4: "Shuxu." Huang Hui, ed., *Lunheng jiaoshi*, vol. 1 (Taipei: Shangwu Yinshuguan, 1983), 174.

104. In contemporary Western practice, acupuncture points are usually identified by the name of the *mo* on which the point lies and a number indicating its order among the points of that *mo*, e.g., the Large Intestine 11 point. However, in classical Chinese nomenclature, this same point was known as the "pond at the bend" (*quchi*). More generally, all the points traditionally had specific names.

What is notable about these names is that they frequently refer to features of the earth's topography. Thus we have ravines (*xi*) and valleys (*gu*), mountains (*shan*) and hillocks (*qiu*), and then a series of terms relating to bodies of water: marshes (*ze*), springs (*quan*), ponds (*chi*), and seas (*hai*). At various places the *mo* are described as emerging (*chu*), passing (*jing*), and entering (*ru*). The image conjured up is of a diverse terrain given unity by the waters that meander through it.

105. This is also true for the so-called *jingmo*, a term often synonymous with the *mo*. The *Suwen* (39/111) thus declares, for instance: "The *mo* flows along and does not stop, circulating without cease."

106. Ozanam, *Circulation*, 483.

107. *Suwen* 28/86; *Lingshu* 38/372. On the importance of the analogy to hydraulic engineering, see the excellent article by Kanō Yoshimitsu, "Isho ni mieru kiron," in Onozawa Seiichi et al., eds., *Ki no shisō* (Tokyo: Tokyo Daigaku Shuppankai, 1978), 281–313 (esp. 289–94). Also see Lu and Needham, *Celestial Lancets*, 22–23; Joseph Needham, *Clerks and Craftsmen in China and in the West* (Cambridge: Cambridge University Press, 1970), 291.

108. *Lingshu* 74/454.

109. *Lingshu* 4/276. See also *Nanjing* 13.

110. *Suwen* 28/86.

111. *Suwen* 18/54.

112. *Suwen* 18/56.

113. *Lingshu* 73/451.

114. *Suwen* 28/86.

115. Kenneth J. DeWoskin, trans., *Doctors, Diviners, and Magicians of Ancient China: Biographies of Fang-shih* (New York: Columbia University Press, 1983), 75.

CHAPTER TWO: THE EXPRESSIVENESS OF WORDS

1. Jean Jacques Menuret de Chambaud, "Pouls," in *Encyclopédie, ou dictionnaire raisonné des sciences, des arts et des métiers* (Facsimile of edition of 1751–80. Stattgard-Bad Canstatt: Friedrich Fromann Verlag, 1966), vol. 13, 222.

2. *Ibid.*, 227.

3. *Ibid.*, 222.

4. *Ibid.*

5. Floyer, *The Physician's Pulse Watch* (London: Samuel Smith and Benjamin Walford, 1707), 232.

6. *Ibid.*

7. *Ibid.*, 355.

8. Stanley Joel Reiser, *Medicine and the Rise of Technology* (Cambridge: Cambridge University Press, 1978), esp. 95–114.

9. Henri Fouquet, *Essai sur le pouls* (Montpellier: Jean Martel, 1767), i.

10. Théophile de Bordeu, *Inquiries Concerning the Varieties of the Pulse, and the Particular Crisis Each More Especially Indicates* (London: T. Lewis and G. Kearsley, 1764), x.

11. James Nihell, *New and Extraordinary Observations Concerning the Prediction of Various Crises by the Pulse*, 2d. ed., (London: John Whiston, Lockyer Davis, John Ward, 1750), iv–vi.

12. Duchemin de l'Etang, "Lettre sur la doctrine du pouls," *Journal de médecine, de chirurgie, et de pharmacie* 29 (1768): 436–39.

13. Milo L. North, "The Proper Influence of the Pulse in Its Applications to the Diagnosis and Prognosis of Diseases," *New England Journal of Medicine and Surgery* 15 (1826): 338–39.

14. Richard Burke, "What are the Practical Indications of the Pulse in Disease?" *London Medical Gazette* 20 (1837), 48–9.

15. Vivian Nutton, *Galen on Prognosis* (Berlin: Akademie-Verlag, 1979), 221; C.R.S. Harris, *Heart and Vascular System* (Oxford: Clarendon Press, 1973) 253.

16. Galen, *Peri diaphoras sphygmōn* 2.1 (K.8.567): "They argue with each other over terms, paying no attention to the realities, and in this way they challenge us with insolent pride and laugh at us if we do not use their terms."

Linguistic competition can be discerned in other fields as well. One Egyptian hermetic writer observes that the meaning of his text, "will become completely obscure when the Greeks take it into their heads to translate it from our language into theirs, which will result in complete distortion and obscurity. Expressed in its original language, however, this discourse retains the meaning of words in all their clarity. In fact, the particularity of the sound and the proper intonation of the Egyptian words preserve in themselves the force of the things one says." (Cited in Pierre Grimal, ed., *Hellenism and the Rise of Rome*, vol. 6 [New York: Delacorte Press, 1968], 217.)

17. G.W. Bowerstock, *Greek Sophists in the Roman Empire* (Oxford: Clarendon Press, 1969), chap. 5, "The Prestige of Galen." Galen himself pleads that he argues against his will. He doesn't want to plod through tedious terminological disputes, he apologizes, but his contemporaries leave him no choice. Whereas the ancients spoke straightforwardly and sought only to transmit their thoughts, rhetoricians now quibble gleefully over every syllable, revel in fatuous cleverness. Frustrated by the impossibility of ignoring this trend, Galen repeats again and again: he argues over definitions only because he must (*Peri diaphoras sphygmōn* K.4.707, 717, 719–20).

18. Cited in Oswei Temkin, *Galenism: The Rise and Decline of a Medical Philosophy* (Ithaca, NY, and London: Cornell University Press, 1973), 181.

19. Bordeu, *Inquiries Concerning the Varieties of the Pulse*, xii–xiii.

20. William Heberden, "Remarks on the Pulse," *Medical Transactions of the Royal College of Physicians* 5 (1772): 18–20.

21. R. Vance, "The Doctrine of the Pulse — an analysis of its character, and summary of its indications," *Cincinnati Lancet and Observer* 26 (1878): 363.

22. Qi De's *Waike jingyi*, for instance, added "long" and "short," which brought the total number of qualities to twenty-six (*YBQS*, 2132–35); Li Shizhen (1518–91) further appended "stiff," bringing the number to twenty-seven (*Pinhu moxue*: *YBQS*, 2140–46); and Li Zhongzi (1588–1655) included "swift" (*Zhenjia zhengyan*: *YBQS*, 2146–64), rounding out a list of twenty-eight qualities, which subsequently became the common standard.

A modern textbook on diagnostic techniques in Chinese medicine compiled in 1972 by the Guangdong Chinese Medicine Institute thus lists twenty-eight varieties of *mo* (*Zhongyi zhenduanxue* [Shanghai: Shanghai Renmin Chubanshe]). Some Qing physicians would include even more qualities. See, e.g., Lin Zhihan, *Sizhen juewei* (Hong Kong: Wanye Chubanshe, n.d.).

23. Author's preface, cited in Taki Gen'in, *Chūgoku isekikō* (Taipei: Dashin Shuju, 1975), vol. 1, 269. For similar comments by Sun Guangyu and Li Shizhen, see also pp. 279 and 287.

24. Wang Shuhe, *Mojing* (Hong Kong: Taiping Shuju, 1961), 1.

25. Li Zhongzi, *Yizong bidu* (Sanyutang edition, 1774), "Mo you bu ke yan-chuan zhi shuo," juan 2, 17a–b.

26. *Ibid.*

27. See, e.g., *Zhuangzi*, juan 1, "Qiwu lun."

28. As the Confucian Xunzi (298–238 B.C.E.) saw the situation in his time: "Men are careless in abiding by established names, strange words come into use, names and realities become confused, and the distinction between right and wrong has become unclear. Even the officials who guard the laws or the scholars who recite the classics have all become confused." (*Hsün Tzu*, chap. 22, "Rectifying Names," trans. Burton Watson, *Basic Writings of Mo Tzu, Hsün Tzu, and Han Fei Tzu* [New York: Columbia University Press, 1964], 141).

29. *Liji*, juan 13, "Wangzhi" (vol. 1, 259).

30. For a careful and balanced discussion of the social contexts shaping the contestation and transmission of knowledge in ancient Greece and China, see G.E.R. Lloyd, *Adversaries and Authorities: Investigations into Ancient Greek and Chinese Science* (Cambridge: Cambridge University Press, 1996). For medicine in particular, also see G.E.R. Lloyd, "Epistemological Arguments in Early Greek Medicine in Comparativist Perspective," and Nathan Sivin, "Text and Experience in Classical Chinese Medicine," in Don Bates, ed., *Knowledge and the Scholarly Medical Traditions* (Cambridge: Cambridge University Press, 1995), 25–40; 177–204, and Bates's introduction to the book. Suggestive comparisons also appear in Nakayama Shigeru, *Academic and Scientific Traditions in China, Japan, and the West*, trans. Jerry Dusenbury (Tokyo: Tokyo University Press, 1984), 3–16.

31. Heinrich von Staden, "Science as Text, Science as History," in Ph.J. van der Eijk et al. eds., *Ancient Medicine in its Socio-Cultural Context*, vol. 2 (Amsterdam and Atlanta: Rodopi, 1995), 511.

32. *Peri diaphoras sphygmōn* 3.7 (K.8.692).

33. M. Ryan, "On the Science of the Pulse," *London Medical and Surgical Journal* 50 (1832): 780.

34. *Peri diaphoras sphygmōn* 3.1 (K.8.638).

35. *Peri diaphoras sphygmōn* 3.1–2 (K.8.644–47).

36. *Peri diaphoras sphygmōn* 2.3 (K.8.574–75).

37. *Peri diaphoras sphygmōn* 1.1 (K.8.496–97); 2.3 (K.8.569); 2.5 (K.8.588); 3.1 (K.8.637ff).

38. *Peri diaphoras sphygmōn* 3.4 (K.8.667); 3.6 (K.8.682); 4.1 (K.8.697).

39. Théophile de Bordeu, *Recherches sur le pouls par rapport aux crises* (Paris, 1754), in *Oeuvres complètes de Bordeu*, with preface by M. le Chevalier Richerand (Paris: Caille et Ravier, 1818), 261.

40. Temkin, *Galenism*, 181.

41. François Nicolas Marquet, *Nouvelle Méthode facile et curieuse pour connoître le pouls par les notes de la musique* (Amsterdam, 1769). These are just a few of the prominent works in a literature that is quite extensive. For a detailed examination of the theme of pulse and music, particularly in the Middle Ages and the Renaissance, see the excellent study by Werner Friedrich Kümmel, *Musik und Medizin: Ihre Wechselbeziehungen in Theorie und Praxis von 800 bis 1800* (Freiburg and Munich: Karl Alber, 1977), chap. 1, "Puls und Musik," 23–62.

42. Cited by Ibn Jumay, *Treatise to Salāh ad-Dīn on the Revival of the Art of Medicine*, ed. and trans. Harmut Fähndrich (Wiesbaden: Deutsche Morgenländische Gesellschaft, 1983), 23.

43. On rhythm, see *Peri diaphoras sphygmōn* 1.8 (K.8.515), on musical training, *Synopsis peri sphygmōn* 12 (K.9.463).

44. Charles Daremberg and Charles Emile Ruelle, eds., *Oeuvres de Rufus d'Ephèse* (Amsterdam: Adolf M. Hakkert, 1963; reprint of the 1879 Paris edition), 224–25.

45. Pliny, *Natural history* 29.4. Galen (*Peri diaphoras sphygmōn* K.8.871) defended Herophilus against this charge, but he himself lodged a similar complaint against Herophilus' followers. Menuret de Chambaud ("Pouls," 220–221) thought enough of Marquet's work to review it at length, but while conceding an undeniable relationship between pulse movements and music, he declared the details of Marquet's renderings "almost without foundation and useless." Still, J.L. Formey reports (*Versuch einer Wurdigung des Pulses* [Berlin: Rucker, 1823], 3) that Marquet's ideas "found not a few followers."

46. Pedro Lain Entralgo, *The Therapy of the Word in Classical Antiquity* (New Haven and London: Yale University Press, 1970), 78. For a thoughtful review of the recent anthropological research on the role of music in healing see Arthur Kleinman, *Writing at the Margin: Discourse Between Anthropology and Medicine* (Berkeley: University of California Press, 1995), 215–22.

47. Edward A. Lippman, *Musical Thought in Ancient Greece* (New York and London: Columbia University Press, 1964), 90.

48. *Philebus* 17c–e; trans. from Lippman, *Musical Thought*, 100.

49. All the references to R. Hackforth's translations are from his *Plato's Examination of Pleasure: A Translation of the Philebus* (Cambridge and New York: Cambridge University Press, 1945).

50. *Philebus* 16c–d (Hackforth's translation found in Edith Hamilton and Huntington Cairns, eds., *The Collected Dialogues of Plato* [Princeton, NJ: Princeton University Press, 1973], 1092).

51. *Laws* 665a: "Order in movement is called rhythm; order in voice — in the blending of the acute with the grave — harmony. The combination of the two is called choric art (*choreia*)." Also *Laws* 669d, 672e; *Symposium* 187c,d; *Gorgias* 502c; *Republic* 397b. Aristotle, *Poetics* 1: "The imitative medium of dancers is rhythm alone, unsupported by music, for it is by the manner in which they arrange the rhythms of their movements that they represent men's characters and feelings and ac tions."

52. Lippman, *Musical Thought*, 53; Thrasybulos Georgiades, *Greek Music, Verse, and Dance* (New York: Merlin Press 1956).

53. In what follows I am indebted to the excellent and concise discussion of the etymology and early uses of *rhythmos* in J.J. Pollitt, *Ancient View of Greek Art* [student edition] (New Haven: Yale University Press, 1974), 135–142.

54. *Histories* 5.58.

55. *Metaphysics* 985b16. The definition is repeated in 1042b14.

56. Diodorus Siculus, *Library of History*, 1.97; Diogenes Laertius, *Lives and Opinions of Eminent Philosophers* 8.47.

57. Pollitt, *Ancient View*, 136–43.

58. Pollitt, *Ancient View*, 138–39. Petersen's original article, "Rhythmus,"

appeared in *Abhandlungen der Königlich Gesellschaft der Wissenschaften zu Göttingen, Philologisch-historische Klasse.* N.F. 16 (1917): 1–104.

59. Werner Jaeger, *Paideia: The Ideals of Greek Culture,* trans. Gilbert Highet, 2d ed., vol. 1 (Oxford: Oxford University Press, 1965), 126.

60. Aristoxenus refers to the divisions within a foot as "signs," or *semeia* (Louis Laloy, *Aristoxène de Tarente, Disciple d'Aristote, et de la Musique de l'Antiquite* [Paris: Société Française d'Imprimerie et de Librairie, 1904], 292 fr. 19). Laloy (298) explains that this was because the chorus director indicated the forms or positions which had to be executed at each of them; and in fact Aristoxenus himself uses *semeion* in the same sense of form (*Aristoxène,* 278 fr. 9).

61. Galen, *Synopsis* 12 (K.9.463f; translation from Harris, *Heart and Vascular System,* 187).

62. *Peri prognōseōs sphygmōn* 2.3 (K.9.278); *Peri diaphoras sphygmōn* 1.25 (K.8.500).

63. *Peri diaphoras sphygmōn* 1.8 (K.8.516).

64. R. Westphal, *Aristoxenus von Tarent: Melik und Rhythmik des classischen Hellentums* (Hildesheim: Georg Olms Verlagsbuchhandlung, 1965), Fragment 6. Laloy, *Aristoxène,* 292.

65. Kümmel, *Muzik und Medizin,* chap. 1.

66. *Mojing,* 2–3.

67. *Mojing,* 4.

68. *Analects* 2.5–7. (Translation from Wing-Tsit Chan, *Source Book in Chinese Philosophy* [Princeton, NJ: Princeton University Press, 1963], 23).

69. Li Gao, *Shishu,* "Bian mo fu suo zhu bing butong" (*YBQS,* 2128); Li Zhongzi, *Yizong bidu,* "Siyan mojue," juan 2, 5b; Li Shizhen, *Pinhu moxue,* "Fu mo" (*YBQS,* 2140).

70. *Suwen* 18/57.

71. Floyer, *Physician's Pulse Watch,* 345.

72. Hua Tuo, *Zhongzang jing* 10 (Taipei: Ziyou Chubanshe, 1986), 10.

73. *Suwen* 17/50.

74. *Analects* 16.7.

75. We catch hints of the importance of subjective sensitivity to *qi* in the

acupuncture technique of Hua Tuo. The *Sanguo zhi* reports that: "He would insert the needle, saying, 'Now I am guiding the qi to this and this place. Tell me when the sensation is felt in that and that place.'" The patient would report the sensations, and as soon as that was done Tuo would withdraw the needle and the disorder would be eliminated. (Kenneth J. DeWoskin, trans., *Doctors, Diviners, and Magicians of Ancient China: Biographies of Fang-shih* [New York: Columbia University Press, 1983], 141; romanization altered.)

76. *Analects* 8.4.

77. *Mencius* 2A.2 (trans. James Legge, *The Works of Mencius* [New York: Dover, 1970], 191).

78. Hua Shou, *Zhenjia shuyao*, "Mo gui you shen" (*YBQS*, 2117).

CHAPTER THREE: MUSCULARITY AND IDENTITY

1. Cited in A. Hyatt Mayor, *Artists and Anatomists* (New York: Artists Limited Edition, 1984), 10.

2. Mayor, *Artists*, 50.

3. Mayor, *Artists*, 10.

4. Mayor, *Artists*, 46. See also Leonardo:

You will make the rule and the measurement of each muscle and give the reason of all their uses, in which manner they work and what moves them, etc.

First make the spine of the back; then clothe it step by step with each of these muscles, one upon the other, and put in the nerves, arteries and veins to each individual muscle; and in addition to this, note to how many vertebrae they are attached, and which intestines are opposite to them and which bones and other organic instruments.... (Charles D. O'Malley and J.B. de C.M. Saunders, *Leonardo da Vinci on the Human Body* [New York: Greenwich House, 1982], 70.)

5. G.E.R. Lloyd, *Magic, Reason and Experience: Studies in the Origins and Development of Greek Science* (Cambridge: Cambridge University Press, 1979), 163.

6. On Diocles, see Werner Jaeger, *Diokles von Karystos* (Berlin: Walter de

Gruyter, 1938), and Fridolf Kudlien, "Problem um Diokles von Karystos," *Sudhoffs Archiv* 47 (1963): 456–64.

7. Ludwig Edelstein, "The History of Anatomy in Antiquity," in *Ancient Medicine*, eds. Owsei and C. Lilian Temkin (Baltimore: Johns Hopkins University Press, 1967), 292.

8. A synopsis of the main arguments can be found in Edelstein's article, "The Development of Greek Anatomy," *Bulletin of the History of Medicine* 3 (1935): 235–48. For a refinement of Edelstein's analysis, see Fridolf Kudlien, "Antike Anatomie und menschlicher Leichnam," *Hermes* 97 (1967): 78–94. James Longrigg has reviewed the problem more recently in "Anatomy in Alexandria in the Third Century B.C.," *British Journal for the History of Science* 21 (1988): 455–88.

A notable exception to the focus on human dissection is G.E.R. Lloyd, "Alcmaeon and the Early History of Dissection," *Sudhoffs Archiv* 59 (1975): 113–47.

9. One of the most interesting analyses of the cultural beliefs surrounding the skin and its trangression appears in Heinrich von Staden, "The Discovery of the Body: Human Dissection and Its Cultural Contexts in Ancient Greece," *Yale Journal of Biology and Medicine* 65 (1992): 223–41.

10. On Homeric medicine, see Charles Daremberg, "La Médecine dans Homère," *Revue Archéologique* n.s. 12 (1865): 95–111; 249–65; 338–55. On the possibility of a Hippocratic anatomy, see Edelstein, "The Development of Greek Anatomy," 251–56; and Lloyd, *Magic, Reason and Experience*, 146ff.

11. Erwin Ackerknecht, *A Short History of Medicine,* rev. ed. (Baltimore: Johns Hopkins University Press, 1982), 14. Evans-Pritchard cites an informant who says: "Azande think that witchcraft is inside a man. When they used to kill a man in the past, they cut open his belly to search there for a witchcraft-substance. If witchcraft-substance was in the belly, they said that the man was a witch. Azande think that witchcraft-substance is a round thing in the small intestine." (*Witchcraft, Oracles and Magic among the Azande* [Oxford: Clarendon Press, 1937], 41.)

12. Ackerknecht, *Short History*, 31.

13. Auguste Bouché-Leclerc, *Histoire de la divination dans l'antiquité,* vol. 1 (Paris: Ernest Leroux, 1879), 166–74; William Reginald Halliday, *Greek Divination* (London: Macmillan, 1913), 186–204.

14. Plato, *Timaeus* 71a–e. The Akkadians connected dissection and prophecy so closely that they used the same word for "flesh" and "omen." They foresaw that a usurper would seize power from the king if the sheep's entrails resembled the face of Humbaba, a demon who lived among "steep climbs" and "barred paths" in the depths of a vast forest, like the Minotaur in the midst of his labyrinth. See François Lenormant, *La Divination et la science des présages chez les Chaldéens* (Paris: Maisonneuve, 1875), 59–60.

15. Bouché-Leclerc, *Histoire,* 170–73.

16. See, e.g., Xenophon, *Anabasis* 6.4.16, 19; 7.6.44; Plutarch, *Lives* 18 ("Cimon") and 73 ("Alexander").

17. Thus Lloyd notes that "The infrequency of dissection for purposes of research is all the more striking in that in another, divination by the inspection of entrails or haruspicy, animals were regularly opened and their parts examined" and suggests that "the contrast in the context and aims of divination, and those of anatomical studies, were no doubt sufficiently marked to act as an effective barrier to communication" (*Magic, Reason and Experience,* 157 n. 165).

Those interested in anatomy, however, were able to profit from the opportunities afforded by sacrifices. See Aristotle, *History of Animals* 496b24ff and *Parts of Animals* 667b1ff.

18. I take Greek hieroscopic divination as just one example. I do not mean thereby to assimilate it with other forms of autopsy such as the Azande search for witchcraft-substance, or even Babylonian haruspicy. Indeed, I take it that there are many forms of autopsy, as different from each other as they are from what we recognize as anatomy, and the study of each of these forms would constitute a worthwhile endeavor. My concern here, however, is just to point out the necessity of understanding the particular form of autopsy that is called anatomy.

19. On the superiority of divination based on animal over human autopsy, see Philostratus, *The Life of Apollonius of Tyana* 8.7 (Loeb ed., vol. 2 [Cambridge, MA: Harvard University Press, 1989] 344–47).

20. Cited in Erwin Ackerknecht, "Primitive Autopsies and the History of Anatomy," *Bulletin of the History of Medicine* 13 (1943): 339n.

21. Ackerknecht, "Primitive Autopsies," 338.

22. Bruno Snell, *The Discovery of the Mind in Greek Philosophy and Literature*, trans. T.G. Rosenmeyer (New York: Dover, 1982), 13.

23. Paul Friedlander, *Plato: An Introduction*, trans. Hans Meyerhof (Princeton, NJ: Princeton University Press, 1969), 13.

24. Kurt von Fritz, *Philosophie und sprachlicher Ausdruck bei Democrit, Plato, und Aristoteles* (New York: G.E. Stechert, 1939), 41–52. C.M. Gillespie reviews the use of these terms in early medical writings in "The Use of Eidos and Idea in Hippocrates," *Classical Quarterly* 6 (1912): 179–203.

25. Plato, *Republic* 517b–c:

> If you interpret the upward journey and the contemplation of things above as the upward journey of the soul to the intelligible realm, you will grasp what I surmise since you were keen to hear it. Whether it is true or not only the god knows, but this is how I see it, namely that in the intelligible world the Form of the Good is the last to be seen, and with difficulty; when seen it must be reckoned to be the cause of all that is right and beautiful, to have produced in the visible world both light and the fount of light, while in the intelligible world it is itself which produces and controls truth and intelligence, and he who is to act intelligently in public or private must see it.

26. Celsus, *De medicina,* "Prooemium," paras. 23ff. (Loeb ed. vol. 1 [Cambridge, MA: Harvard University Press, 1971], 12–14).

27. Celsus, *De medicina*, "Prooemium," paras. 27ff; Karl Deichgraber, *Die griechische Empirikerschule*, 2d. ed. (Berlin: Weidmannsche Verlagsbuchhandlung, 1965), 130–32 and 281ff.

28. Rufus of Ephesus, *De corporis humani partium appellationibus* 9 (Daremberg and Ruelle, 134).

29. *History of Animals* 1.16, 494b21f.

30. Charles Singer, trans., *Galen on Anatomical Procedures* (London: Oxford University Press, 1956), 34.

31. Singer, *Anatomical Procedures*, 34–35.

32. Singer, *Anatomical Procedures*, 33–34.

33. Galen, *Peri chreias tōn moriōn* Book 10.12 (K.3.812–13).

34. Preface to *De humanis corporis fabrica*, translated in the appendix to C.D. O'Malley's *Andreas Vesalius of Brussels, 1514–1564* (Berkeley: University of California Press, 1964), 323.

35. Jaeger, *Diokles*, 165. On Erasistratus, see Galen, *Peri dynameōn physikōn* 2.2 (K.2.78). For a good example of how teleological thinking shaped Aristotle's anatomy see Simon Byl, "Note sur la place et la valorisation de la ΜΕΣΟΤΗΣ dans la biologie d'Aristote," *L'Antiquité Classique* 37 (1968): 467–76.

36. G.E.R. Lloyd, *Hippocratic Writings* (Reading: Penguin, 1978), 349. No consensus, however, has been reached on the dating of this text, and many have argued for a post-Aristotelian dating. See I.M. Lonie, "The Paradoxical Text on the Heart," *Medical History* 17 (1973): 2

37. The classic treatment of teleology is Willy Theiler, *Zur Geschichte der teleologischen Naturbetrachtung bis auf Aristoteles* (Zurich and Leipzig: Orell Füssli, 1925). Friedrich Solmsen discusses the craftsman image in "Nature as Craftsman," *Journal of the History of Ideas* 24 (1963): 473–96.

38. *Phaedo* 97c.

39. Xenophon, *Memorabilia* 1.4.

40. *Gorgias* 503e.

41. *Republic* 10.596b.

42. *Timaeus* 29a.

43. *Phaedo* 99d–e.

44. *Phaedo* 79c–d. For some of the countless other instances of this opposition of sense and intellect in Plato, see *Timaeus* 27d ff, and *Philebus* 59c.

45. Plato, *Republic* 7.533d. See Friedlander, *Plato*, 13. For further examples of similar expressions in Plato, see Theodor Gomperz, *Apologie der Heilkunst: Eine griechische Sophistenrede des fünften vorchristlichen Jahrhunderts*, Zweite Auflage (Leipzig: Verlag von Veit, 1910), 155.

46. It is worth noting that, in the Hippocratic treatise *Peri archaiēs iatrikēs* (22–23), the author stresses the importance of studying the internal structures

(*schēmata*) of the body by appealing to the connection between their forms (*eidea*), i.e., their shape, and their functions (e.g., a broad hollow body that tapers is best suited for attracting fluid).

47. Solmsen, "Nature as Craftsman," 490.

48. *Metaphysics* 7.8. Of course, even in this Aristotelian interpretation, "Form" meant much more than it does for us. Form was inseparably fused with function, and this not necessarily in a mechanical way, as we might imagine the connection, but *qua* form. Thus in the *History of Animals* (1.7) Aristotle notes with respect to the shape of the forehead that "Persons who have a large forehead are sluggish, those who have a small one are fickle, those who have a broad one are excitable, those who have a bulging one, quick-tempered."

49. See, e.g., *Physics* 193a and 198b. On form and function and *technē*, see *Generation of Animals* 734b34ff and 740b25ff.

50. *Parts of Animals* 645a.

51. *Parts of Animals* 644b.

52. Singer, *Anatomical Procedures*, 5 and 77.

53. *Peri chreias tōn moriōn* 3.3 (translation from Arthur J. Brock, *Greek Medicine* [London: J.M. Dent & Sons, 1929; New York: AMS Press, 1979], 155).

54. Thus Edmund Dickinson remarks: "[T]he knife and lectures of a skilful anatomist, cannot but preach religion even to the very atheist, when he sees the stupendous make of living creatures, when he considers the subtility, the variety, and wise contrivance of parts in the most minute, as well as in the largest animals..." (preface to John Browne, *Myographia nova, or a Graphical Description of All the Muscles in Humane Body as They Arise in Dissection* [London, 1697]).

55. In the *Orator*, Cicero makes parallel observations about the apperception of beauty in art:

> But I do believe that there is nothing in any genre so beautiful that that from which it was copied, like a portrait of a face, may not be more beautiful; this we cannot perceive either with eyes or ears or any other sense, but we comprehend it without our mind and with our thoughts; thus we can imagine things more beautiful than Phidias's sculptures, which are the most beautiful we have seen in their genre ...; and indeed, that artist,

when he produced his Zeus or his Athena, did not look at a [real] human being whom he could imitate, but in his own mind there lived a sublime notion of beauty; this he beheld, on this he fixed his attention, and according to its likeness he directed his art and hand. (Cited in Erwin Panofsky, *Idea: A Concept in Art Theory*, trans. Joseph J.S. Peake [New York: Icon Editions, 1968], 12.)

56. Singer, *Anatomical Procedures*, 149.

57. *Peri agmōn* 2 and 4 (L.3.422, 428). See also Aristotle, *Parts of animals* 2.8.

58. *Peri kardiēs* 4 (L.9.82).

59. *Peri kardiēs* 6 (L.9.84).

60. *Peri trophēs* 51 (L.9.118). The passage does go on to observe that the exercised parts (*ta gegymnasmena*) — note the passive form — are more resistant to change; but it makes no suggestion that the muscles are any more actively engaged in exercise than bones.

61. Galen, *Peri myōn anatomēs* (K.18.926). Lycus' *Peri myōn* was supposedly the first monograph devoted entirely to muscles.

62. Galen, *On the Doctrines of Hippocrates and Plato*, ed., trans., and commentary by Phillip de Lacy, pt. 1, bks. 1–4 (Berlin: Akademie Verlag, 1981 [2d ed.]), 99.

63. *Physiognomics* 810a15–31.

64. Sophocles, *Women of Trachis* 1103.

65. Euripides, *Orestes* 228.

66. *Generation of Animals* 732a26–27; see also 774b13–14.

67. *Peri gonēs* 18 (L.7.504).

68. Sophocles, *Oedipus the King* 718. See also *Women of Trachis* 779.

69. *Oedipus the King* 1270. Later Aristotle would explain why the eyes were the last part of the body to become articulated. *Generation of Animals* 744b10–12.

70. Oribasius, *Collectiones medicae* 8.38 (Ioanes Raeder, ed., *Oribasii collectionum medicarum reliqiae*, vol. 1 [Leipzig: B.G. Teubner, 1928], 289).

71. See, e.g., Aristotle, *Generation of Animals* 748b25–26 and *History of Animals* 504b22–23. Also Herodotus 3.87 and 4.2.

72. Aristotle, *Rhetoric to Alexander* 1435a35; see also *Poetics* 1457a6.

73. *History of Animals* 535a30–31.

74. *History of Animals* 536a1–3.

75. Strabo, *Geography* 14.2.28.

76. *Diodorus* 3.17 (Trans. C.H. Oldfather, *Diodorus of Sicily*; Loeb Classical Library [Cambridge, MA: Harvard University Press, 1935]).

77. Diodorus, 3.18.3.

78. Diodorus, 3.18.5–6.

79. *Parts of Animals* 667a9–10.

80. *Peri aerōn, hydatōn, topōn* 19 (L.3.70–72; trans., slightly modified, from W.H.S. Jones, *Hippocrates*, vol. 1; Loeb Classical Library [Cambridge, MA: Harvard University Press, 1972], 123). On the moistness of the constitution and environment of the Scythians, see also Aristotle, *Generation of Animals* 5.3.

81. *Peri aerōn, hydatōn, topōn* 20 (L.2.74; trans. Jones, *Hippocrates*, 123–25).

82. The regimen of top contemporary bodybuilders includes eight hours of weightlifting and nine pounds of meat (not to mention other foods, protein supplements, and pills) *per day*. See Charles Gaines, *Pumping Iron: The Art and Sport of Bodybuilding* (New York: Simon and Schuster, 1974).

83. *Aphorismoi* 1.3 (L.4.460).

84. *Republic* 3.404a.

85. *Republic* 3.410c–d.

86. *Republic* 3.411a–b.

87. *Republic* 3.411e–412a.

88. Herodotus, *Histories* 9.121. Trans. Aubrey de Sélincourt, *Herodotus: The Histories* (Harmondsworth: Penguin, 1976), 624.

89. *Peri aerōn, hydatōn, topōn* 24 (L.2.86–88; trans. Jones, *Hippocrates*, 137).

90. *Peri aerōn, hydatōn, topōn* 23 (L.2.82–86; trans. Jones, *Hippocrates*, 133). Here climatic influences are accentuated by differences in government. Ruled by kings, Asian "souls are enslaved, and refuse to run risks readily." By contrast, the independent Europeans "are willing and eager to go into danger, for they themselves enjoy the prize of victory."

91. *Peri gonēs* 18 (L.7.504).

92. *Peri diaitēs* 8 (L.6.484–5).

93. *Physiognomics* 810a15–31.

94. *Peri aerōn, hydatōn, topōn* 22 (L.2.80–82).

95. *Peri aerōn, hydatōn, topōn* 21 (L.2.74–76).

96. *Problems* 894b20–21.

97. Galen, *Peri myōn kinēseōs* 1.1 (K.4.367). The definition opens the work.

98. *Peri myōn kinēseōs* 2.4 (K.4.435ff).

99. *Peri myōn kinēseōs* 2.5 (K.4.440ff).

100. *Peri myōn kinēseōs* 1.8 (K.4.404–6).

101. Jean-Pierre Vernant, "Dim Body, Dazzling Body," *Zone 3: Fragments for a History of the Human Body*, eds. Michel Feher, Ramona Naddaff, and Nadia Tazi (New York: Zone Books, 1989), 29.

102. Albrecht Dihle thus notes that the Homeric term *menos* comes "indeed very near to the modern notion of will," but adds that *menos* "does not belong to the normal or natural equipment of man according to Homeric psychology." It comes from the gods, as "an additional gift, provided only on a special occasion and not supposed to become a lasting part of the person..." (*The Theory of Will in Classical Antiquity* [Berkeley: University of California Press, 1982], 34).

We may recall, in a related vein, how Homer's Agamemnon blames his tragedy not on any personal decisions or actions, but on *atē*, a distinctly impersonal clouding of the mind. E.R. Dodds (*The Greeks and the Irrational* [Berkeley: University of California Press, 1951], 15–16) interprets this not as a self-justifying evasion, but as a reflection of the fact that the Homeric Greeks had no concept of a unified personality. Bruno Snell, to whom Dodds refers, famously argued, indeed, that the Greeks in Homer's time didn't even "yet have a body in the modern sense of the body," did not, that is, "know it *qua* body, but merely as the sum total of his limbs." (*The Discovery of the Mind in Greek Philosophy and Literature* [New York: Dover, 1982; German edition, 1948], 6–8). For a critique of Snell's position see Bernard Knox, *The Oldest Dead White European Males* (New York: W.W. Norton, 1993), 37–41.

103. Daremberg and Ruelle, *Rufus*, 184.

104. *Movement of Animals* 11 and 7.

105. Galen, *Doctrines of Hippocrates and Plato*, 99.

106. *History of Animals* 536b5–7. (Trans. A.L. Peck, Aristotle, *History of Animals Books IV–VI*; Loeb Classical Library [Cambridge, MA: Harvard University Press, 1970], 81–83).

107. *Generation of Animals* 744a33–744b9.

108. For discussion of this issue, see the essays in Mary Louise Gill and James G. Lennox, eds., *Self-motion: From Aristotle to Newton* (Princeton, NJ: Princeton University Press, 1994); and Martha Craven Nussbaum, *Aristotle's De motu animalium* (Princeton, NJ: Princeton University Press, 1978).

109. Georges Canguilhem, *La Formation du concept de réflexe aux XVIIe et XVIIIe siècles* (Paris: Librairie Philosophique J. Vrin, 1977), 16.

110. *Peri myōn kinēseōs* 1.3 (K.4.377); *Peri anatomikōn encheirēseōn* 7.8 (K.2.610). Admittedly, his rejection of the heart's muscularity does not rely entirely on function. He goes on in the same passage to suggest that the substance of muscles is softer and redder than what one finds in the heart, and that the heart tastes different than muscles, especially when boiled.

The modern interpretation of the heart as a muscle dates back only to 1664, when the Danish anatomist Nicholas Steno, in *De musculis et glandulis observationen specimen*, uncoupled the notion of muscle from the theme of voluntary motion. In this work, Steno propounded his famous axiom, *cor vere musculus est*, and argued that "in the heart nothing is lacking of that which is in a muscle, and nothing is in it which is not also in a muscle." See E. Bastholm, *The History of Muscle Physiology: From the Natural Philosophers to Albrecht von Haller* (Copenhagen: Ejnar Munksgaard, 1950), 145.

111. On Herophilus' views of the voluntary character of the nervelike parts, see Galen, *Peri tromou kai palmou kai spasmou kai rigous* 5 (K.7.605–6); on the involuntary nature of the pulse, see Rufus, *Synopsis peri sphygmōn* 2 (Daremberg and Ruelle, 220–21), and von Staden, *Herophilus*, 255–56. Galen remarks similarly, "The motions of the arteries and veins are natural (*physikai*) and occur without the will, whereas those of the muscles are psychic (*psychikai*) and follow from the will." (*Peri myōn kinēseōs* 1.1 [K.4.372])

112. Galen, *Doctrines of Hippocrates and Plato*, 81.

113. Galen, *Doctrines of Hippocrates and Plato*, 123.

114. Galen, *Doctrines of Hippocrates and Plato*, 99.

CHAPTER FOUR: THE EXPRESSIVENESS OF COLORS

1. *Nanjing* 61.

2. *Lingshu* 4/275.

3. *Shanghanlun*, juan 1, 19a.

4. *Shiji*, chap. 105 (vol. 6, 2785). For an acute analysis of the available evidence about Bian Que, see Yamada Keiji, "Henjaku densetsu," *Tōhō gakuhō* 60 (1988): 73–158.

5. See, e.g., Stephen A. Tyler, "The Vision Quest in the West, or What the Mind's Eye Sees," *Journal of Anthropological Research* 40 (1984): 23–40.

6. For a review of references to dissections in China, see Watanabe Kōzō, "Genzon suru Chūgoku kinsei made no gozō roppu zu no gaisetsu," in his *Honzō no kenkyū* (Osaka: Takeda Kagaku Shinkōkai, 1987), 341–452.

A. Hyatt Mayor (*Artists and Anatomists* [New York: Artists Limited Edition, 1984], 3) observes, "Even after some Chinese had begun modern dissection in the early nineteenth century, most Chinese continued to have vague notions of anatomy, for Yu Li-tch'ou then said that missionaries would give up and go home if they had the sense to realize that they could never convert a people like the Chinese whose hearts grow on the right side. The only Chinese who could be Christianized were the few freaks whose hearts grew on the left like barbarians."

7. The *Lingshu* passage does reappear in treatise 3 of the *Taisu*, but this is due to the close genetic connection between these two texts and does not really represent a third reference. I should point out that the passage in the Wang Mang biography is the *sole* mention of dissection to be found in any the official histories (*zhengshi*) that so voluminously document Chinese history. Medical sources, however, make clear that dissections did occur in later periods.

8. *Hanshu* 69b (vol. 5, 4145–46). The translation for this and other passages cited in this section of the chapter are drawn from the article by Yamada Keiji, "Anatometrics in Ancient China," *Chinese Science* 10 (1991): 39–52. This article summarizes arguments presented at greater length in Yamada's article in Japa-

nese: "Hakkō-ha no keiryō kaibōgaku to jintai keisoku no shisō," in Yamada Keiji and Tanaka Tan, eds., *Chūgoku kodai kagakushi ron* (*Zokuhen*) (Kyoto: Kyoto Daigaku Jimbun Kagaku Kenkyūjo, 1991): 427–92. While the ultimate thrust of these articles concerns the history of the composition of the *Huangdi neijing*, they are also important contributions to the history of Chinese anatomy.

9. Mikami Yoshio, "Omō jidai no jintai kaibō," *Nihon ishigaku zasshi* (1943): 1–28.

10. *Shiji*, chap. 3 (vol. 1, 108).

11. *Lingshu* 12/311.

12. On the agreement between these figures and the archaeological evidence of cadavers excavated from Han tombs, see Yamada, "Hakkō-ha no keiryō kaibōgaku."

13. *Lingshu* 14/319–20.

14. *Lingshu* treatises 31 and 32/359–62; *Nanjing* 42 and 43. For a more detailed review of classical Chinese "anatometrics" and translations of many of the relevant passages, see Yamada, "Anatometrics."

15. Yamada, "Anatometrics," 52.

16. *Lingshu* 14/319.

17. Yet another way to cut open the body and look is exemplified by Mesopotamian haruspicy. See Jean Bottéro, "Symptōmes, signes, écritures, en Mésopotamie ancienne," in Jean-Pierre Vernant et al., *Divination et rationalité* (Paris: Editions du Seuil, 1974), 70–193.

18. Max Simon, *Sieben Bücher Galeni* (Berlin, 1906) vol. 2, vii.

19. *Nanjing* 1.

20. *Suwen* 8/28.

21. *Suwen* 23/76.

22. *Shiji*, chap. 105 (vol. 6, 2793). A variant of the same episode is recounted in the *Hanfeizi*, chap. 21, "Yu lao" (juan 7, 2b–3a).

23. *Suwen* 5/23.

24. *Suwen* 5/23.

25. *Lingshu* 59/417.

26. *Suwen* 18/55.

27. Since the *Nanjing* was composed as a commentary on the difficulties of the *Neijing*, it is unlikely that this technique of differential pressures represented a *Nanjing* innovation. The same technique appears in a portion of the *Shanghan-lun* ("Pingren mofa," juan 1, 21b) attributed to Wang Shuhe, where it is introduced by the header *jingshuo*, "The classic says...." The method doesn't appear, however, in the extant recensions of the *Neijing*.

28. *Suwen* 39/113; *Lingshu* 49/401. Sometimes, black is deemed to mean something different from green. See *Suwen* 56/151 and *Lingshu* 74/455.

29. *Suwen* 32/94.

30. The color-phase correspondences ran as follows:

phase	wood	fire	earth	metal	water
color	green	red	yellow	white	black

31. For instance, one might compare the tinge of the face as a whole with the hue tinging the white of the eyes. See *Suwen* 10/36.

32. *Shiji*, chap. 4 (vol. 1, 120).

33. *Shiji*, chap. 6 (vol. 1, 237–38).

34. *Shiji*, chap. 60 (vol. 4, 2115). See also the commentary to the *Shujing* "Yu gong" (juan 6, 6b).

35. *Suwen* 13/41–42.

36. *Suwen* 10/36.

37. Thus in the biography of Hua Tuo in the *Sanguo zhi* (see Kenneth J. DeWoskin, *Doctors, Diviners, and Magicians of Ancient China: Biographies of Fang-shih* [New York: Columbia University Press, 1983], 140–53), the great doctor reaches his diagnosis most often by palpation, and we are told that "he cured disorders by feeling the pulse, and his results could be likened to that of a spirit" (DeWoskin, 147). However, the biography also makes clear the possibility of diagnosing just from the face: "Yan Xin, who was a native of Yandu, was waiting with his retinue of men to see Tuo. As soon as Tuo appeared, he questioned Xin: 'Are things well inside you?' Xin replied, 'I am the same as always.' But Tuo went on to warn him, 'You have a severe disorder. I can see it in your face. Do not drink too much wine' (DeWoskin, 142; romanization altered)."

38. *Suwen* 13/42.

39. *Nanjing* 13.

40. *Suwen* 5/23.

41. Chunyu Yi's biography, I noted, emphasizes the pulse. Nonetheless, observation of *se* still forms part of his practice. A book on the *mo* tops the list of texts that his master transmits to him; but listed second is a work on color diagnosis. See *Shiji*, chap. 105 (vol. 6: 2794, 2796, 2807).

42. *Mencius* 7B.24 (trans. D.C. Lau, *Mencius* [Harmondsworth: Penguin, 1970], 198).

43. See, e.g., *Zhuangzi*, chap. 12 (juan 5, 11a).

44. These include the *Shujing* (Zhou shu, "Hong fan"), *Zuozhuan* (Duke Zhao, years 20 and 25), and *Zhuangzi* (chaps. 8, 9, 12). However, all the extant versions of these texts include later interpolations, so that the mere appearance of a phrase doesn't guarantee the use of the term at the time of the text's original composition. The literature on the evolution of five-phase analysis is extensive. See, e.g., Xu Fuguan, *Zhongguo renxinglun shi. Xian Qin bian* (Taizhong: Donghai University, 1963); A.C. Graham, *Yin-yang and the Nature of Correlative Thinking* (Singapore: Institute of East Asian Philosophies, 1986).

45. *On the Soul* 2.7.

46. *Liji*, juan 6, "Tangong I" (vol. 1, 113).

47. Nakajima Yōsuke, *Goshiki to gogyō. Kodai chūgoku tenbyō* (Tokyo: Bon Books, 1986), 89.

48. *Analects* 16.6 (trans. D.C. Lau, *Confucius: The Analects* [Harmondsworth: Penguin, 1979], 140).

49. *Analects* 10.3.

50. *Mencius* 1A.4; 3B.9.

51. *Mencius* 1B.1

52. *Zhuangzi*, chap. 18 (juan 6, 18b); chap. 20 (juan 7, 9a).

53. See Tōdō Akiyasu, ed., *Kanwa daijiten* (Tokyo: Gakushū Kenkyūsha, 1978), 619. Tōdō also points out etymological connections to terms such as *mu*, "longing (for what is not there)," and *mu*, "to recruit (to fill a vacancy)."

54. *Zhuangzi*, chap. 29 (juan 9, 21a, 24a).

55. *Analects* 9.18; 15.13.

56. *Mencius* 4A.4.

57. *Liezi* (juan 8, 3): "Those whose beauty is in the prime (*sesheng zhe*) are proud"; *Zhanguoce*, juan 14, "Strategems of Chu (pt.1) 10 (vol. 2, 719).

58. *Shujing*, Zhou shu, "Tai zhe (pt.1) (juan 11, 2b); *Mencius* 1B.5; *Liji*, juan 51, "Fangji" (vol. 2, 870–71): "The gentleman distances himself from lust (*se*) and establishes himself as a model for the people."

59. *Shujing*, Zhou shu: "Jiong ming" (juan 19, 8b).

60. *Analects* 1.3; 17.17. See also 5.25.

61. *Analects* 12.20; 17.10.

62. *Shujing*, Yu shu: "Gao yao mo" (juan 4, 10b).

63. *Lunheng*, chap. 79 (vol. 2, 1089–91).

64. *Ibid.*, 1091–92.

65. The intimate ties between *wangqi* and military concerns are detailed in chaps. 4 and 5 of Sakade Yoshinobu's, *Chūgoku kodai no sempō* (Tokyo: Kembun Shuppan, 1991), 128–83.

66. Onozawa Seiji, Fukunaga Mitsuji, Yamanoi Yū, eds., *Ki no shisō* (Tokyo: Tokyo Daigaku Shuppankai, 1978), 154–56; 183–84; 230.

67. "[The diviner] Zi Shen gazed into the atmosphere and prophesized: 'This year there will be turmoil in Song, and the state will nearly perish. Things will settle down after three years. There will be soon be a catastrophe in Cai'" (*Zuozhuan*, Duke Zhao year 20 [juan 25, vol. 3, 1209]).

68. *Shiji*, juan 27, "Tianguan shu" (vol. 3, 1336–37).

69. *Houhan shu*, "Mingdi ji."

70. *Lingshu* 4/275. The *Yitong guayan* remarks that "The magpie (*que*) is a yang bird. It anticipates things and moves. It anticipates events and responds." Interestingly, this word *que* (i.e., magpie) is the same character that appears in the name Bian Que.

71. *Lingshu* 49/401. In the *Shiji* (juan 7, "Xiang Yu benji," vol. 1, 311) a diviner gazes upon the *qi* of Liu Bang and sees a tiger and dragon glowing with the five colors — the aura of a true Son of Heaven. See Sakade, 156–57.

72. *Mencius* 7A.38.

73. *Analects* 12.20 (trans. Lau, *Confucius*, 116).

74. *Mencius* 2A.2 (trans. James Legge, *The Works of Mencius* [New York: Dover, 1970], 191).

75. *Boran bianse*: *Mencius* 5B.9; also 1B.1: "the king blushed" (*wang bian hu se*). *Boran zuose*: *Zhuangzi*, chap. 12 (juan 5, 10a). See also *Analects* 10,3: "When he (Confucius) was summoned by his lord to act as his usher, his face took on a serious expression (*se boru ye*)." *Fenran zuose*: *Zhuangzi*, chap. 12 (juan 5, 7a). *Furan zuose*: *Zhuangzi*, chap. 12 (juan 5, 10a).

76. *Zhuangzi*, chap. 3 (juan 5, 7b). The translation is from Burton Watson, trans., *The Complete Works of Chuang Tzu* (New York: Columbia University Press, 1968), 135.

77. *Analects* 8.4 (trans. Lau, *Confucius*, 92).

78. *Analects* 2.8 (trans. Lau, *Confucius*, 64).

79. *Analects* 8.2.

80. *Zhuangzi*, chap. 19 (juan 7, 3b); see also chap. 6 (juan 3, 7a).

81. *Sanguo zhi*, "Hua Tuo zhuan." See DeWoskin, *Doctors, Diviners, and Magicians*, 140 and 150.

82. *Iliad* 13, lines 278–84; 19, lines 38–39; 21, lines 567–68; 24, lines 413–14.

83. Galen, *Peri ton symptōmatōn diaphoras* 1.1 (K.7.44).

84. Elizabeth C. Evans, *Physiognomics in the Ancient World*, in *Transactions of the American Philosophical Society*, new series, vol. 59 (Philadelphia: American Philosophical Society, 1969), 14.

85. *Lingshu* 10/305.

86. *Shujing*, Zhou shu: "Bi ming" (juan 19, 4a); *Chunqiu Gongyang zhuan*, Duke Huan, year 2.

87. *Suwen* 17/50; 81/254; 10/34.

88. *Lingshu* 10/305.

89. *Lingshu* 4/275.

90. *Nanjing* 8. This explains how it can happen that a person with an ostensibly healthy pulse suddenly dies. It is as in the case of plants: when the roots are suddenly cut, the plant may, judged by the flowers and leaves, initially seem fine.

91. *Shanghanlun*, juan 1, 10b.

92. This view remained strong in postclassical medicine as well. Sun Simiao, for instance, asserts, "The various floating and rootless *mo* indicate death; the five *zang* and six *fu* are the root" (*Qianjin fang*, "Zhen wuzang liufu qijue zhenghou" [*YBQS*, 2441]). The Jin dynasty physician Liu Wansu maintained that only by matching voices and colors can a diagnostician determine "the flowering or withering of the *zang* and the *fu*" (*Liu shu*, "Chase lun" [*YBQS*, 2441]). Zhu Zhenheng: "The five colors are the flower of *qi*; responding to the five phases and matching the four seasons, they appear in the face" (*Xinfa*, "Neng he se mo keyi wanquan" [*YBQS*, 2444]).

93. *Suwen* 10/34. See also *Suwen* 17/50.

94. *Zhanguoce*, juan 14, "Strategems of Chu (pt. 1)" 10 (vol. 2, 719); *Shiji*, "Lu Buwei liezhuan" (vol. 5, 2507–8).

95. John Ruskin, *Queen of the Air: Being a Study of the Greek Myths of Cloud and Storm* (New York: Hurst and Company, n.d.; preface dated 1869), 96–7.

96. Galen, *Peri dynameōn physikōn* 1.1 (K.2.1)·

97. "But in ensuing time, as all the organs become even drier, not only are their functions performed less well but their vitality becomes more feeble and restricted. And drying more, the creature becomes not only thinner but also wrinkled, and the limbs weak and unsteady in their movements. This condition is called old age, and is analogous to the withering of plants; for that is likewise the old age of a plant, arising from excessive dryness. This, then, is one innate destiny of destruction for every mortal creature" (Robert Montraville Green, trans., *Galen's Hygiene* [Springfield, MA: Charles C. Thomas, 1951], 7).

98. *Mencius* 2A.2 (translation from D.C. Lau, *Mencius* [London: Penguin, 1970], 78). For other important uses of the plant analogy, see also *Mencius* 6A.8. 9.

99. *Suwen* 81/254.

100. *Guoyu*, juan 11, "Jinyu." For flower as *se*: *Hanshu*, juan 27C, "Wuxing zhi" (vol. 3, 1442); *Mencius* 7A. 21.

101. Derk Bodde, *Chinese Thought, Society, and Science: The Intellectual and Social Background of Science and Technology in Pre-modern China* (Honolulu: Univer-

sity of Hawaii Press, 1991), 311. Ho's remarks appear in his *The Cradle of the East: An Inquiry into the Indigenous Origins of Techniques and Ideas of Neolithic and Early Historic China, 5000–1000 B.C.* (Hong Kong: Chinese University of Hong Kong, and Chicago: University of Chicago Press, 1975), 113–14.

CHAPTER FIVE: BLOOD AND LIFE

1. Galen, *Peri phlebotomias therapeutikon* 10 (K.11.281).

2. Galen, *Peri phlebotomias pros Erasistraton* 1 (K.11.147–48).

3. "Bloodletting at prescribed intervals for the healthy, or as a form of urgent treatment for the sick, was certainly the commonest form of medical intervention in the Middle Ages" (Peter Murray Jones, *Medieval Medical Miniatures* [London: The British Library, 1984], 119).

4. Cited in Lynn Thorndike, *A History of Magic and Experimental Science During the First Thirteen Centuries of our Era* (New York: Columbia University Press, 1923), vol. 1, 728.

5. From his letter to a learned physician, for instance, we learn of how the Abbot of Cluny (d. 1156) was phlebotomized on a regular, bimonthly basis, and became extremely worried when a variety of circumstances forced him to miss his scheduled treatment. See Nancy Siraisi, *Medieval and Early Renaissance Medicine: An Introduction to Knowledge and Practice* (Chicago: University of Chicago Press, 1990), 115–16.

6. Cited in Peter Niebyl, "Galen, van Helmont and Blood Letting," in A.G. Debus, ed., *Science, Medicine and Society in the Renaissance*, vol. 2 (New York: Science History Publications, 1972), 18.

7. Lorenz Heister, *A General System of Surgery in Three Parts*, 7th ed. (London, 1759), 273.

8. Marshall Hall, *Principle of the Theory and Practice of Medicine* (Boston: Charles C. Little and James Brown, 1839), 203. Cited in Leon S. Bryan, "Bloodletting in American Medicine, 1830–1892," *Bulletin of the History of Medicine* 38 (1964): 518.

9. Charles Waterton, *Natural History: Essays* (London: Frederick Warne, 1871), 42–43.

10. To be sure, enthusiasm for phlebotomy was never universal or unqualified. Even in antiquity there were skeptics: Chrysippus the Cnidian, for example, shunned the practice, as did his renowned disciple Erasistratus (K.11.151).

11. The passage is cited and translated by Peter Brain in his *Galen on Bloodletting: A Study of the Origins, Development and Validity of His Opinions*, with a translation of the three works (Cambridge: Cambridge University Press, 1986), 112.

12. Brain, *Galen on Bloodletting*, 118–19. Littré was not alone in his view of Hippocratic bloodletting. Haeser, for instance, in his *Geschichte der Medizin* (1845), maintained that Hippocrates resorted to phlebotomy in all feverish diseases, especially when dealing with young, strong people. (See Bauer, *Geschichte der Aderlass*, 17 n. 4. In the note, however, Bauer criticizes the unfounded nature of Haeser's assertion.)

13. Celsus, *De medicina* 2.10.1.

14. Yamada Keiji, "Shinkyū to tōeki no kigen. Kodai Chūgoku igaku keisei no futatsu no isō," in Yamada, ed., *Shin hatsugen Chūgoku kagakushi shiryō no kenkyū. Ronkō hen* (Kyoto: Kyoto Daigaku Jimbun Kagaku Kenkyūjo, 1985): 3–122.

15. Maruyama Masao, *Shinkyū igaku to koten no kenkyū* (Osaka: Sōgensha, 1977), 60–61.

16. D.C. Epler, "Bloodletting in Early Chinese Medicine and Its Relation to the Origin of Acupuncture," *Bulletin of the History of Medicine* 54 (1980): 337–67.

17. *Taiping guangji*, juan 218.

18. Gao Wu, *Zhenjiu juying*, juan 2, "Dongyan zhenfa" and "Lifeng" (Taipei: Hongye Shuju, 1974), 160–63 and 178.

19. On bloodletting and leprosy, see Suzuki Noriko, *Nihon kinsei shakai to yamai — rai igaku no tenkai o megutte*, Ph.D. diss., Graduate University for Advanced Studies, Kyoto, 1997. For bleeding in *sha* disorders, see Guo Zhisui, *Shazhang yuheng* (1675).

20. Günther Lorenz's *Antike Krankenbehandlung in historischvergleichender Sicht* (Heidelberg: Carl Winter Universitätsverlag, 1990) also deals at length

with ancient bloodletting from a comparative perspective. Because Lorenz's analysis of Greek bloodletting concentrates on Hippocrates, however, his book doesn't address the main questions with which this chapter deals. His discussion of Chinese bloodletting relies mostly on Epler.

21. Aeschylus, *Eumenides* 251ff; Leviticus 17.14.

22. Niebyl, "Galen, van Helmont and Blood Letting," 14–15. William Harvey, however, all while acknowledging the association of blood and life, decried the rejection of bloodletting: "Now when I maintain that the living principle resides primarily and principally in the blood, I would not have it inferred from thence that I hold all bloodletting in discredit as dangerous and injurious; or that I believe with the vulgar that in the same measure as blood is lost, is life abridged, because the sacred writings tell us that the life is in the blood" (cited in Niebyl, 18).

23. *Suwen* 10/35.

24. *Analects* 16.7.

25. *Suwen* 62/168. This passage goes on to prescribe bloodletting for excess blood.

26. *Iliad* 18, line 110; G.S. Kirk and J.E. Raven, *The Presocratic Philosophers* (Cambridge: Cambridge University Press, 1964), 344. Natural philosophers, according to Aristotle (*On the Soul* 403a–b), link the surging of blood and heat around the heart with anger.

27. *Peri hiērēs nousou* 11.

28. *Pros Erasistraton* 5 (K.11.165–66).

29. *Suwen* 62/167.

30. Blood could not only determine a person's qualities, but could identify that person as someone *of* quality: "Of this generation and blood do I claim to be," Glaukos maintains proudly in the *Iliad* (6, line 211; see also 20, line 241).

31. Galen, *Peri phlebotomias pros Erasistrateious tous en Romē* 4 (K.11.212).

32. Galen, *Tōn pros Glaukōna therapeutikōn* 1.15 (K.11.53). Also *Pros Erasistrateious tous en Romē* 4 (K.11.218–20) and *Phlebotomias therapeutikōn* 1 (K.11.251).

33. *Phlebotomias therapeutikōn* 1 (K.11.251).

34. *Aphorismoi* 6.36.

35. *Peri tōn entos pathōn* 28 and 32 (L.7.242, 251).

36. *Peri physios anthrōpou* 10.

37. *Peri hiērēs nousou* 6; *Peri physios anthrōpou* 2; *Peri osteōn physios* 9; *Peri topōn tōn kata anthrōpon* 3; *History of Animals* 3.2.511b. Marie-Paule Duminil provides a detailed review of the various accounts of the *phlebes* and the interrelations between them in *Le Sang, les vaisseaux, le coeur dans la collection Hippocratique* (Paris: Société d'Édition "Les Belles Lettres," 1983), 15–131.

38. Peter Brain, for instance, approvingly cites J. Mewalt's disparaging comment on Hippocrates' "strange account of vasculature" (*wunderliche Aderbeschreibung*) (Brain, *Galen on Bloodletting*, 114). Mewalt's article is "Galenos bei echte und unechte Hippocratica," *Hermes* 44 (1905): 111–34.

39. On the idea of circulation in Chinese medicine see Lu Gwei-djen and Joseph Needham, *Celestial Lancets: A History and Rationale of Acupuncture and Moxa* (Cambridge: Cambridge University Press, 1980), 24–39.

40. *Suwen* 63/173.

41. *Suwen* 41/117.

42. Epler's article, "Bloodletting in Early Chinese Medicine," for instance, defends this thesis.

43. *Peri aerōn, hydatōn topōn* 10.

44. There are a few exceptions. For example, Peter Brain suggests, tentatively, and with many qualifications, one possible benefit that bloodletting may have had. Citing studies relating changes in blood chemistry and susceptibility to infection, he notes that copious bloodletting lowers the iron level in the blood, and that this in turn may have reduced the ability of certain bacteria to reproduce (*Galen on Bloodletting*, 158–72). On the possible effectiveness of bloodletting to fight fevers, see Norman W. Kasting, "A Rationale for Centuries of Therapeutic Bloodletting: Antipyretic Therapy for Febrile Diseases," *Perspectives in Biology and Medicine* 33.4 (1990): 509–15.

45. Charles Rosenberg highlights this last factor, pointing to the professional usefulness of a remedy like bloodletting, which produced fairly dramatic and predictable effects, and thus showed the patient that the doctor's cure was

"working." See "The Therapeutic Revolution," in Morris J. Vogel and Charles E. Rosenberg, eds., *The Therapeutic Revolution: Essays in the Social History of American Medicine* (Philadelphia: University of Pennsylvania Press, 1979), 8.

46. *Medieval Medical Miniatures*, 121.

47. *Pros Erasistrateious tous en Romē* 4 (K.11.212; 218–20); *Phlebotomias therapeutikōn* 1 (K.11.251).

48. "The idea that one should simply let blood from patients who are at risk of a plethos," he observes, "is not yet worthy of Hippocrates' art."

> I should prefer to have explained to me the manner in which the evacuation should be effected, and on what occasion, and to what extent. To establish when one should cut the vein in the forehead, and when those at the corners of the eyes, or under the tongue, the one known as the shoulder vein, or the one through the axilla, or the veins in the hams, or alongside the ankle, concerning all of which Hippocrates taught — this, I think, is the proper study of physicians (*Pros Erasistrateious tous en Romē* 6 [K.11.168–69] = Brain, *Galen on Bloodletting*, 28).

See also *Phlebotomias therapeutikōn* 11 [K.11.283–84]; 15 [K.11.295–96]).

49. In the Middle Ages, indeed, topological bleeding was given special prominence by the associations of particular bleeding sites with particular astrological signs. See Loren McKinney, *Medical Illustrations in Medieval Manuscripts* (London: Wellcome Historical Medieval Library, 1965), 55–56. On medieval debates about the significance of which side of the body one bled from, see Pedro Gil-Sotres, "Derivation and Revulsion: The Theory and Practice of Medieval Phlebotomy," in Luis García-Ballester et al., eds., *Practical Medicine from Salerno to the Black Death* (Cambridge: Cambridge University Press, 1994).

50. See, for instance, book 2 of his *Therapeutics of Acute Diseases* (Francis Adams, trans. and ed., *The Extant Works of Aretaeus the Cappadocian* [London: Sydenham Society, 1856], 422–23).

51. Thus, while praising the humoral doctrines propounded in the *Peri physios anthrōpou*, Galen rejected its descriptions of the vessels as a later interpolation; so obviously false anatomically, it could not reflect the teaching of the great Hippocrates. (*Peri tōn Hippokratous kai Platōnos dogmatōn* 6.3 [K.5.529].)

52. See, e.g., *Pros Erasistrateious tous en Rom̄e* 4 (K.11.218–19 = Brain, *Galen on Bloodletting*, 53): "Some say that it makes no difference which vein one chooses to cut, since the whole body can be evacuated equally well through any of them; others, however, take the contrary view that there is a very great difference, since some veins evacuate the affected part quickly, others in a longer time."

53. The remarks of Saunders and O'Malley on the context of Vesalius' *Venesection Letter* of 1539 remind us that the influence did not just flow from anatomy to phlebotomy:

> Galenic physiology and notions based upon it engendered an abnormal preoccupation with the venous system, and with the publication of the *Venesection Letter* and further Vesalian studies, this preoccupation became intensified. One need only examine an anatomical work appearing after the middle of the sixteenth century to observe the disproportionate treatment given to the venous over the arterial system — a complete reversal of what obtains in the modern textbook — to appreciate how deeply the physician was concerned with its every detail.... At our distance we are apt to forget that venesection was the major practical therapeutic measure.... Its effective exploitation depended upon knowledge of the venous system ... (John B. de C.M. Saunders and Charles Donald O'Malley, *Andreas Vesalius Bruxellensis: The Bloodletting letter of 1539* [New York: Henry Schuman, 1947], 19).

Saunders and O'Malley further describe in this work how controversies about the relationship between phlebotomy and anatomical structure contributed to the development of anatomy.

54. *Pros Erasistraton* 6 (K.11.169 = Brain, *Galen on Bloodletting*, 28).

55. *Ibid.*, 168.

56. For the following discussion of Hippocratic material I am much indebted to the excellent dissertation of Peter Niebyl, *Venesection and the Concept of a Foreign Body: A Historical Study in the Therapeutic Consequences of Humoral and Traumatic Concepts of Disease* (Ph.D. diss., Yale University, 1969).

57. *Epidēmiōn* 1. The translation is from W.H.S. Jones, trans., *Hippocrates,*

vol. 1, Loeb Classical Library (Cambridge, MA: Harvard University Press, 1972), 171.

58. *Ibid.*, 167. In keeping with the topological consciousness of Hippocratic physicians, reports of nosebleeds routinely specify whether the bleeding occurred in the left nostril, the right nostril, or both.

59. *Epidēmiōn* 6.3.23 (L.5.304).

60. *Kōakai prognōsies* 2.15 (L.5.649).

61. *Kōakai prognōsies* 6.31 (L.5.702). On menstruation and conceptions of the female body in Hippocratic writings, see Leslie Dean-Jones, *Women's Bodies in Classical Greek Science* (Oxford: Clarendon Press, 1994), 86–109.

62. *Epidēmiōn* 4.58 (L.5.196).

63. *Peri helkōn* 2 (L.6.402–4).

64. *Peri nousōn* 4.38 (L.5.554–57). The equation of food and blood remained stable through antiquity. Aristotle summarizes matters with characteristic succinctness. "It is plain," he says, "that blood is the final form of food in animals that have blood.... This explains why the blood diminishes in quantity when no food is taken, and increases when it is; and why, when the food is good, the blood is healthy, and when bad, poor" (*Parts of Animals* 2.3.650a–b).

65. *Peri topōn tōn kata anthrōpon* 43 (L.6.336–37).

66. *Phlebotomias therapeutikon* 8 (K.11.276).

67. *Phlebotomias therapeutikon* 8 (K.11.273); *Therapeutikēs methodou* 8.4 (K.10. 564–67).

68. *Therapeutikēs methodou* 4.6 (K.10,287ff); *Hippokratous peri diaitēs okseōn nosematōn biblion kai Galēnou hypomnēma* 4.17 (K.15,766); *Hippokratous to peri arthrōn biblion kai Galēnou eis auto hypomnēmata* 3.64 (K.18A,575–6).

69. *Phlebotomias therapeutikon* 8 (K.11.273).

70. *Pros Erasistrateious tous en Romē* 8 (K.11.237).

71. Some of Galen's contemporaries apparently believed that Erasistratus had phlebotomized. Galen argues at length against this belief in *On Venesection Against the Erasistrateans at Rome.*

72. *Pros Erasistrateious tous en Romē* 8 (K.11.236). For more on the Erasistratean theory of plethoric inflammation, see J.T. Vallance, *The Lost Theory of*

Asclepiades of Bithynia (Oxford: Clarendon Press, 1990), 126–30.

73. Much of *On Venesection Against Erasistratus* is devoted to just this point. See especially *Pros Erasistraton* 4 (K.11.156–57) and 8–9 (K.11.172–86).

74. Galen regularly speaks of bleeding as a form of "evacuation," thus relating it with defecation and micturition. After urging the self-evident necessity of evacuating a *plethos* of blood, for example, he goes on: "What, after all, is the assimilation of nutriment but the establishment of a *plethos*? and what is defecation but the evacuation of the overloaded bowel? What is micturition if not a cure for the full bladder?" (*Pros Erasistraton* 6 [K.11.167] = Brain, *Galen on Bloodletting*, 27–28)

75. *Phlebotomias therapeutikon* 3 (K.11.257–58).

76. *Peri kriseōn* 2.12 (K.9.693).

77. Even in the latter half of the nineteenth century Charles Waterton (*Natural History*, 42) still averred, "I consider inflammation to be the root and origin of all diseases. To subdue this at its earliest stage has been my constant care." This was why he had regularly had himself bled — prophylactically, to prevent inflammation.

78. L.J. Rather, *The Genesis of Cancer: A Study in the History of Ideas* (Baltimore: Johns Hopkins University Press, 1978), 13.

79. Rather, *Genesis*, 11.

80. Robert Montraville Green, trans., *Galen's Hygiene* (Springfield: Charles C. Thomas, 1951), pt. 6, chap. 6, 251.

81. *Peri diaphoras pyretōn* 1.6 (K.7.290–91).

82. For a discussion of the notion of seeds of disease in antiquity and afterward, see Vivian Nutton, "The Seeds of Disease: An Explanation of Contagion and Infection from the Greeks to the Renaissance," *Medical History* 27 (1983): 1–34.

83. *Peri diaphoras pyretōn* 2.15 (K.7.384–87).

84. *Therapeutikēs methodou* 6.2 (K.10.386–87).

85. *Peri plēthous* 1 (K.7.515–16).

86. *Phaedrus* 248c.

87. *Phaedo* 81c.

88. Rudolph Arbesmann, "Fasting and Prophecy in Pagan and Christian Antiquity," *Traditio* 7 (1949–51): 3.

89. Philostratus, *Life of Apollonius* 8.5; 8.7; cf. 2.37.

90. Cited in Herbert Musurillo, "The Problem of Ascetical Fasting in the Greek Patristic Writers," *Traditio* 12 (1956): 13. For more on the relationship between food and spirituality, see the fascinating study by Caroline Bynum, *Holy Feast and Holy Fast: The Religious Significance of Food to Medieval Women* (Berkeley: University of California Press, 1987).

91. Zhou Yimou and Xiao Zuotao, eds., *Mawangdui ishu kaozhu* (Taipei: Loqun wenhua shiye youxian gongsi, 1989), 228.

92. Sima Qian, *Shiji*, chap. 55 (vol. 4, 2048).

93. *Lingshu* 81/480; 66/438.

94. *Lingshu* 60/419.

95. *Zhuangzi* 13, "Tiandao" (juan 5, 12a).

96. *Suwen* 5/22. This echoes *Zhuangzi* 20 ("Shanmu" [juan 7, 106]): "Who can harm the person who wanders the world abiding in emptiness?"

97. *Suwen* 5/22.

98. *Suwen* 1/7. I have slightly modified the translation from Nathan Sivin, *Traditional Medicine in Contemporary China* (Ann Arbor, MI: Center for Chinese Studies, University of Michigan, 1987), 98.

99. *Suwen* 28/86.

100. Revealingly, the earliest use of the *xushi* contrast in any sense approximating its usage in medicine appears in military strategy. In Sunzi's famous treatise on tactics, *xu* and *shi* articulate one of the work's most famous principles. In a chapter entitled *Xushi* (chap. 6), Sunzi explains that one should "avoid [one's enemies when and where they are] *shi*, and attack [them when and where they are] *xu*. Chapter 5 explains *xu* and *shi* by suggesting that the deployment of troops should be like hard stone smashing eggs. It will be evident, however, that this usage of *shi* still differs somewhat from its sense in medicine.

101. *Suwen* 53/145.

102. *Laozi* 77.

103. For more on the techniques and philosophical background of supple-

menting and dispersing in acupuncture, see Murakami Yoshimi, "Kōtei daikei taiso no igaku shisō," in Yamada Keiji, ed., *Chūgoku kodai kagakushi ron* (Kyoto: Jimbun kagaku kenkyūjo, 1989), 3–53.

104. *Lingshu* 1/264.

105. The sages of old, the *Suwen* explains more concretely, taught people to abide in limpidity and empty nothingness, so that the spirit was preserved within and diseases had no room to enter (*Suwen* 1/8).

106. *Lingshu* 66/437. Sivin's translation (*Traditional Medicine*, 100–101), slightly modified.

107. *Zhuangzi* 22, "Zhi bei you" (juan 7, 23a).

108. *Huainanzi* (Taipei: Zhonghua Shuju, 1976), juan 7, 2b–3a.

109. *Hanfeizi* 20 (Chen Qiyou, *Hanfeizi jishe* [Beijing: Zhonghua Shuju, 1958], vol. 1, 326).

110. Green, *Galen's Hygiene*, 53–54.

111. *Pros Erasistraton* 5 (K.11.164).

112. Themison and other Methodists held that menstruation only contributed to childbearing. But they held this position against those who held that menstruation also contributed to health. This latter group, Soranus reports, held that "nature provides for mankind. She recognizes that men rid themselves of surplus matter through athletics, whereas women accumulate it in considerable quantity because of the domestic and sedentary life they lead, and mindful that they ... do not fall into danger, she has provided to draw off the surplus through menstruation" (Owsei Temkin, trans., *Soranus' Gynecology* [Baltimore: Johns Hopkins University Press, 1956], 23).

113. *Generation of Animals* 4.6.775a–b.

114. *Suwen* 40/114. Not surprisingly, therefore, later Chinese writers on menstrual disorders tended to emphasize drugs that replenished and vivified the blood, thus counteracting depletion. See Charlotte Furth, "Blood, Body and Gender: Medical Images of the Female Condition in China," *Chinese Science* 7 (1986), 54–56.

Galen actually distinguished two varieties of fullness. One was *plethos* by filling, a distention of the vessels caused by excess blood — the condition to which purists restricted the term plethora. The other, dynamic *plethos*, was the buildup due to the weakness of the excretory faculty. The latter kind, which made excess a consequence of prior weakness, thus paralleled the dependence, in Chinese medicine, of *shi* on *xu*. But note the divergence in the conceptions of weakness: *xu* was a failure to *retain* vitality; the weakness that led to dynamic *plethos* was a failure to *expel* residues.

115. Galen, *Peri tōn peponthotōn topōn* 6.5 (K.8.416–19). Translation from Rudolph Siegel, *Galen on the Affected Parts* (Basel: S. Karger, 1976), 183–85. On the debilitation, however, that can result from continual loss of sperm, and on the strength that follows from continence, see the discussion of "gonorrhea" in Aretaeus, *On the Causes and Symptoms of Chronic Diseases* 2 (Adams, *Extant Works of Aretaeus*, 346–47).

116. Donald Harper discusses the Mawangdui *fangshu* texts in "The Sexual Arts of Ancient China as Described in a Manuscript of the Second Century B.C.," *Harvard Journal of Asian Studies* 47 (1987): 539–93. The classic discussion of techniques of self-cultivation, including *fangshu*, is Henri Maspéro, "Les Procédés de 'nourrir le principe vital' dans la religion taoiste ancienne," *Journal Asiatique* 229 (1937): 177–252. On the history of Chinese sexual arts more generally, see R.H. van Gulik, *Sexual Life in Ancient China* (Leiden: E.J. Brill, 1961).

117. Sivin, *Traditional Medicine*, 51–52, 147–164.

118. Theophrastus (*De sensu* 39ff) reports Diogenes' theory thus: "Pleasure and pain come about in this way: whenever air mixes in quantity with the blood and lightens it, being in accordance with nature, and permeates through the whole body, pleasure is produced; but whenever the air is present contrary to nature and does not mix, then the blood coagulates and becomes weaker and thicker, and pain is produced. . . ."

119. *Generation of Animals* 2.6.741b.

120. On the "spiritualization" of *pneuma* over the course of antiquity, see Gérard Verbeke, *L'Evolution de la doctrine du pneuma: Du stoicisme à Saint Augustin* (Paris: Desclée De Brouwer, 1945).

121. It should be noted that Hippocratic ideas of the *phlebes*-like Chinese

notions of *mo*, straddled this division of blood vessels and nerves. *Phlebes* carried blood, and this was why they were the objects of phlebotomy; but they also conveyed sensation and governed control of the limbs: blockage of them could result in paresthesia, or paralysis, or spasms. The clear separation of blood vessels from nerves occurred only gradually: Praxagoras, for instance, still thought nerves merely the finest ends of thicker arteries.

122. Galen, *Peri myōn kinēseōs* 1 (K.4.372).

123. Friedrich Solmsen, "The Vital Heat, the Inborn Pneuma, and the Aether," *Journal of Hellenistic Studies* 77 (1957): 119–23; Everett Mendelsohn, *Heat and Life: The Development of the Theory of Animal Heat* (Cambridge, MA: Harvard University Press, 1964).

124. *Timaeus* 70c–d; Aristotle, *On Youth, Old Age, Life and Death, and Respiration* 469b21f; Mendelsohn, *Heat and Life*, 8–26.

125. *Peri diaphoras sphygmōn* 4.2 (K.8.714); *Peri chreias sphygmōn* 3 (K.5.161; Furley and Wilkie, 206).

126. Galen, *Peri chreias sphygmōn* 3 (Furley and Wilkie, 206; K.5.161); *Doctrines of Hippocrates and Plato* 2, 4–5.

127. *Peri chreias sphygmōn* 7.3 (Furley and Wilkie, 221; K.5.173–74).

128. *Peri chreias sphygmōn* 7.4 (Furley and Wilkie, 223; K.5.174–75).

129. *Peri diagnōseōs sphygmōn* 1.3–7 (K.8.786–806).

130. In *Peri prognōseōs sphygmōn* 2.2 (K.9.276), Galen summarized the relationship between pulse size, frequency, heat, and residues as follows:

With respect	increased heat	larger diastole	frequent
to the outer	increased residues	earlier systole	frequent
rest	decreased heat	smaller diastole	rare
	decreased residues	slower systole	rare
With respect	increased residues	longer systole	frequent
to the inner	increased heat	earlier diastole	frequent
rest	decreased residues	smaller systole	rare
	decreased heat	slower diastole	rare

CHAPTER SIX: WIND AND SELF

1. *Epidēmiōn* 1.1 (L.2.598).

2. The role of winds in *Peri diaitēs* is discussed by Carl Fredrich, "Die vier Bucher *Peri diaitēs*," in his *Hippokratische Untersuchungen* (Berlin, 1899; reprint, New York: Arno Press, 1976), esp. 159–67.

3. *Aphorismoi* 3.12 (L.4.490); *Peri aerōn, hydatōn, topōn* 10 (L.2.42–50); *Peri hiērēs nousou* 13 (L.6.384–86).

4. *Peri aerōn, hydatōn, topōn* 1 (L.2.12).

5. *Suwen* 42/120; *Lingshu* 49/400; *Suwen* 3/13.

6. Erwin Ackerknecht, *A Short History of Medicine*, rev. ed. (Baltimore: Johns Hopkins University Press, 1982); Charles Singer and E. Ashworth Underwood, *A Short History of Medicine*, 2d ed. (New York: Oxford University Press, 1962); Henry E. Sigerist, *A History of Medicine*, 2 vol. (Oxford University Press, 1951 [vol. 1] and 1961 [vol. 2]); Arturo Castiglioni, *A History of Medicine*, 2d ed. (New York: Alfred A. Knopf, 1947); Max Neuburger, *History of Medicine* (London, 1910); Fielding Garrison, *Introduction to the History of Medicine*, 4th ed. (Philadelphia: W.B. Saunders, 1929); Benjamin Lee Gordon, *Medicine Throughout Antiquity* (Philadelphia: F.A. Davis, 1949); John Hermann Bass, *Outlines of the History of Medicine and the Medical Profession*, trans. H.E. Handerson (New York: J.H. Vail, 1889).

7. Students of Chinese medicine have, however, considered the problem of wind pathology in the *Neijing*. See notably, Ishida Hidemi, "Kaze no byōinron to chūgoku dentō igaku shisō no keisei," *Shisō* 799 (1991): 105–24, and Paul Unschuld, "Der Wind als Ursache des Krankseins," *T'oung Pao* 68 (1982): 91–131. The main focus of Yamada Keiji's essay "Kyūkyū happū setsu to shōshiha no tachiba" (*Tōhō gakuhō* 52 (1980): 199–242) concerns the formation of the *Huangdi neijing*, but it also includes extensive discussion of classical Chinese wind theory.

8. *Peri aerōn, hydatōn, topōn* 4 and 5.

9. Plato, *Laws* 5.747d.

10. *Hanshu*, juan 28B (vol. 2, 1640). In a related vein, the preface to the *Fengsu tongyi* (preface, 1) observes: "The *feng* [of *fengsu* refers to the fact] that among airs (*tianqi*) some are warm and some cold, among terrains some are

mountainous and some flat, among water sources some are pure and some pol-luted, among trees and grasses some are hard and some flexible." See also *Suwen* 12/39–40 for a discussion of the impact of local geography on health.

11. See Zhuangzi's earlier cited remarks on the "music of the earth," and also *Huainanzi* (juan 6) and Zhang Hua, *Bowu zhi* (juan 8).

12. Hiraoka Teikichi, *Enanji ni arawareta ki no kenkyū* (Tokyo: Risōsha, 1968), 48; Akatsuka Kiyoshi, "Kaze to miko," in his *Chūgoku kodai no shūkyō to bunka* (Tokyo: Kadokawa Shoten, 1977), 442.

13. *Lunheng*, juan 5, "Ganxu" (*Lunheng jiaoshi*, 220); *Lingshu* 75/462. See also *Huainanzi* (juan 7, 2a): "Blood and *qi* are wind and rain."

14. *Antigone* 929–30; Ruth Padel, *In and Out of the Mind: Greek Images of the Tragic Self* (Princeton, NJ: Princeton University Press, 1992), 91.

15. It was Hu Houxuan who initially drew attention to ancient Chinese wind names and the wind spirits governing the four directions ("Jiaguwen sifang fengming kaozheng," in his *Jiaguxue Shangshi luncong*, vol. 2 [Chengdu: Chilu University, 1944], 1–6). Since then, the nature of Shang wind conceptions has been elucidated by Yan Yiping, "Zhongguo yixue zhi qiyuan kaolue," pt. 1, *Dalu zazhi* 2.8 (1951): 20–22, pt. 2, *Dalu zazhi* 2.9 (1951): 14–17; Ding Shan, "Sifang zhi shen yu fengshen," in *Zhongguo gudai zongjiao yu shenhua kao* (Shanghai: Shanghai wenyi chubanshe, 1988), 78–95; Kaizuka Shigeki, "Kaze no kami no hakken," in *Chūgoku no shinwa* (Tokyo: Chikuma Shobō, 1971), 76–109; and Akatsuka Kiyoshi, "Kaze to miko," in his *Chūgoku kodai no shūkyō to bunka* (Kadokawa Shoten, 1977), 415–42.

16. For inscriptional references to winds and hunting, see Akatsuka, "Kaze to miko," 425–27.

17. *Zuozhuan*, Duke Xi year 4. The Han-dynasty dictionary *Shuowen* suggests that the insect radical in the character for wind derives from the fact that insects stir when the wind blows.

18. *Huainanzi*, juan 1, 5b–6a. On the classical and medieval European beliefs about wind as fecundating agent, see Conrad Zirkle, "Animals Impreg-nated by Wind," *Isis* 25 (1936): 95–129.

19. *Huainanzi*, juan 13, 9b.

20. Sakade Yoshinobu, "Kaze no kannen to kaze uranai," in *Chūgoku kodai no sempō. Gijutsu to jujutsu no shūhen* (Tokyo: Kembun Shuppan, 1991), 102–103.

21. *Shiji*, juan 27, "Tianguan shu" (vol. 3, 1340).

22. Wang Chong, *Lunheng* (vol. 1, 650–52).

23. *The Suppliant Women* 549–554. See also Lucretius, *De rerum natura* 5.1226.

24. Aeschylus, *Seven Against Thebes* 707–708.

25. Sophocles, *Oedipus at Colonus* 607–615 (trans. Robert Fitzgerald, in David Grene and Richard Lattimore, eds., *Sophocles I* [Chicago and London: University of Chicago Press, 1954], 107)

26. *Odyssey* 10.1ff.

27. Herodotus, *Histories* 2.77.3. See also Hippocrates, *On Humors* 16.

28. *Analects* 12.19.

29. *Zuozhuan*: Duke Zhao year 20; Duke Yin year 5. See also Duke Xiang year 29: "the five sounds are harmonized, and the eight airs equally [blended]." On the possibility of using music to diagnose changes in wind and rain, see *Huainanzi* (juan 8, 4a). In *Lunheng* 15 (*Lunheng jiaoshi*, 673), *feng* in the sense of song, seems related to the chants that bring rain.

30. *Zuozhuan*, Duke Xiang year 29 (juan 20, vol. 2, 1000–1001). Earlier in the *Zuozhuan* (Duke Xiang year 18; juan 17, vol. 2, 878) the musician Shi Kuang of Jin, after singing songs from both the north and the south, predicts from the relative weakness of the southern airs (*nanfeng*) the failure of an attack launched by the southerly kingdom of Chu.

31. *Lülan*, juan 6, pian 3.

32. *Shijing* "Da xu." Translation modified from James Legge, *The Chinese Classics*, vol. 4, *The She King* (Taipei: Southern Materials Center, 1985), pt. 1, p. 35. The association of winds, politics, and the power of indirect persuasion also appears in *Analects* 12.19, quoted above.

33. Sir John Davis thus translates *Guofeng* as "Manners of the different states." ("The Poetry of the Chinese," *Transactions of the Royal Asiatic Society*, May 1829; cited in Legge, *The She King*, pt. 1, p. 2, n. 1). In that article Davis cites a passage from the *Spectator* (no. 502): "I have heard that a minister of state

in the reign of Queen Elizabeth had all manner of books and ballads brought to him, of what kind soever, and took great notice of how much they took with the people; upon which he would, and certainly might, very well judge of their present dispositions, and of the most proper way of applying them according to his own purposes"(Legge, "Prolegomena," 23).

34. Cited in the *Hanshu*, juan 28B (vol. 2, 1640). By the same token, immoral songs could induce immorality. Thus Confucius objected to the lewd songs of Zheng and worried about their pernicious influence on people elsewhere (*Analects* 15.10). In his edition of the *Shijing*, James Legge (*The Chinese Classics*, vol. 4, "Prolegomena," 23) cites "Andrew Fletcher of Saltoun," who relates the opinion of "a very wise man, that if a man were permitted to make all the ballads of a nation, he need not care who should make its laws." The *Fengsu tongyi* (2, 1a) similarly quotes Confucius as teaching that the sage Shun "began by regulating the six tunings, equalizing the five voices, and mastering the eight airs, and thus all the world followed his lead."

35. Burton Watson, *The Complete Works of Chuang Tzu* (New York: Columbia University Press, 1968), 36–37.

36. *Zhuangzi* 22, "Zhi bei you" (juan 7, 23a).

37. *Iliad* 2.536. Richard Broxton Onians, *The Origins of European Thought About the Body, the Mind, the Soul, the World, Time, and Fate* (Cambridge: Cambridge University Press, 1954), 49–56.

38. Padel, *In and Out*, 90.

39. Aeschylus *Suppliant Maidens* 166–67; Euripides, *Ion* 1501–9:

> Fate drove us hard in the past,
> Just now oppressed us again.
> There is no harbor of peace
> From the changing waves of joy and despair.
> The wind's course veers.
> Let it rest. We have endured
> Sorrows enough. O my son,
> Pray for a favoring breeze
> Of rescue from trouble.

The use of *pneuma* to mean breath, however, isn't unknown. Aeschylus, for instance, also evokes a "mare's nostril breath," and Euripides the "sweet breath of children." See *Seven against Thebes* 463 and *Medea* 1074.

40. Padel, *In and Out*, 93–94. See *Electra* 1202; *Andromacha* 610.

41. *Peri physōn* 3 (L.VI, 94).

42. For an interpretation of Greek medicine, however, that attaches considerable importance to this text and to the theory of winds/breaths in general, see Jean Filliozat, *La Doctrine classique de la médecine indienne: Ses origines et ses parallèles grecs* (Paris: Imprimerie Nationale, 1949).

43. *Peri hiērēs nousou* 7 (L.6.372–74).

44. *Peri hiērēs nousou* 16 (trans. G.E.R. Lloyd, *Hippocratic Writings*, 247–48).

45. *Peri chymōn* 17 (L.5.498).

46. Volker Langholf, *Medical Theories in Hippocrates* (Berlin: W. de Gruyter, 1990), 170–77.

47. See *Odyssey* 5.296; *Iliad* 5.524–26.

48. H. Frisk, *Griechisches etymologisches Wörterbuch* 3 Bde (Heidelberg: C. Winter, 1960–70).

49. The pseudo-Aristotelian treatise *The Situation and Names of Winds* (973b) in fact derives *notos* from *nosos* (sickness).

50. Virgil, *Georgics* 1.443–44: "the south wind unkind (*sinistra*) alike to trees and crops and herds."

51. Theophrastus, *De sensu* 39ff (DK 64A 19). Aristophanes (*Clouds* 227) remarks on the effects of different kinds of air on intelligence. See also Stobaeus, *Anthologion* 3.5.7: "A man when he is drunk is led by an unfledged boy, stumbling and not knowing where he goes, having his soul moist"; and 3.5.8: "A dry soul is wisest and best (*auē psychē sophōtatē kai aristē*)."

52. Lazarus Rivière, *The Practice of Physick* (London: George Sawbridge, 1678), 51.

53. Jean Bodin, *Method for the Easy Comprehension of History*, trans. Beatrice Reynolds (New York: Octogon Books, 1966), chap.5, "The Correct Evalution of Histories"; Montesquieu, *The Spirit of the Laws*, bk. 14, "Of Laws in Relation to the Nature of the Climate." For a survey of ideas about the environment and

human being, see Clarence J. Glacken, *Traces on the Rhodian Shore: Nature and Culture in Western Thought from Ancient Times to the End of the Eighteenth Century* (Berkeley: University of California Press, 1967).

54. Yan Yiping, "Zhongguo yixue zhi qiyuan kaolue" (pt. 2), *Dalu zazhi* 2.9 (1951): 15.

55. Miyashita Saburō, "Chūgoku kodai no shippeikan to ryōhō," *Tōhō gakuhō* 30 (1959): 227–52.

56. *Zuozhuan*, Duke Zhao year 1.

57. Another reference to wind and sickness appears in *Mencius* 2B.2, where the king excuses himself from visiting Mencius by saying that he has a cold disease (*hanji*) and thus can't expose himself to the wind. The short Mawangdui treatise "The Avoidance of Grains and the Eating of Breaths," for its part, advises that in the summer one should drink in the morning mist, and avoid drawing in the hot afternoon wind. See Yamada Keiji, ed., *Shin hatsugen Chūgoku kagakushi shiryō no kenkyū. Shakuchū hen* (Kyoto: Kyōto Daigaku Jimbun Kagaku Kenkyū-jo, 1985), 291–96

58. *Lingshu* 66/437; *Suwen* 26/82.

59. For details of the theory of the nine palaces and eight winds as it applied to medicine, see Ishida, "Kaze no byōinron."

60. For early attempts to relate the eight directions and the eight partitions of the year, see the *Huainanzi*, juan 3 and 4.

61. John Major, "Notes on the Nomenclature of Winds and Directions," *T'oung pao* 65 (1979): 66–80. The expression *bafeng* appears already in the *Zuozhuan*, but there it designates not eight winds, but eight tunes or airs.

62. Yamada, "Kyūkyū happūsetu," 206.

63. Yan Guojie, "Guanyu Xihan chuqide shipan he zhanpan, *Kaogu* (1978): 334–37; Yin Difei, "Xihan Ruyinhou mu chutude zhanpan he tenwen yiqi," *Kaogu* (1978): 338–43.

64. *Lingshu* 77/467–69. On the theory of the nine palaces and eight winds, see Ishida, "Kaze no byōin ron"; Yamada, "Kyūkyū happū setsu"; and Shirasugi Etsuo, "Kyūkyū happūzu no seiritsu to Kato Rakusho no denshō," *Nihon Chūgoku gakkai hō* 46 (1994): 16–30.

65. *Huainanzi*, juan 3.

66. *Suwen* 2/10.

67. *Suwen* 4/16.

68. *Suwen* 17/52.

69. *Suwen* 56/152: "Thus the birth of the hundred diseases necessarily begins with the skin and body hair (*mao*). The noxious breaths attack it and the pores open up, the pores open up and [the noxious breaths] enter and occupy the subsidiary conduits; if it remains and isn't eliminated, it transfers and enters the major conduits...." See also *Suwen* 63/172 and *Lingshu* 66/437–38.

70. *Lingshu* 47/393–93.

71. *Lingshu* 47/390.

72. *Lingshu* 50/403.

73. *Suwen* 3/15.

74. *Suwen* 3/13.

75. *Suwen* 35/102.

76. *Galēnou tōn eis to peri chymōn Hippocratous hypomnēmatōn* 3 (K.16,395–411; 438–44).

77. *Peri philosophou historias* 20 (K.19,292); *Hippokratous epidēmiōn A kai Galēnou eis auto hypomnēma* 2.4 (K.17A,90); *Peri euporistōn* 3 (K.14,557); *Peri diagnōseōs sphygmōn* 4.1 (K.8,925); *To Hippokratous kat' iētreion biblion kai Galēnou eis auto hypomnēma* 1.11 (K.18B,684); *Pros Pisōna peri tēs thēriakēs* 11 (K.XIV, 251).

78. In fact, of course, even in the West wind-consciousness was not really a dead end. Later on, *Airs, Waters, Places* still enjoyed much influence. See note 53 above.

79. Gérard Verbeke, *L'Evolution de la doctrine du pneuma: Du stoicism à saint Augustin* (Paris: Desclée De Brouwer, 1945). Other important studies include Max Wellmann, *Die pneumatische Schule bis auf Archigenes in ihrer Entwicklung dargestellt* (Berlin: Weidmannsche Buchhandlung, 1895); Werner Jaeger, "Das Pneuma im Lykeion," *Hermes* 1913: 29–74; and most recently, Armelle Debru, *Le Corps respirant* (Leiden: E.J. Brill, 1996).

80. *Peri diaitēs okseōn* 5 (L.2.406).

81. See Gad Freudenthal, *Aristotle's Theory of Material Substance: Heat and Pneuma, Form and Soul* (Oxford: Clarendon Press, 1995).

82. John 4.24.

83. Frederick Sargent's *The Hippocratic Heritage* (Elmsford, NY: Pergamon Press, 1982) offers a good survey of the history of Western meteorological medicine.

84. Jean-Marie Annoni et Vincent Barras, "La Découpe du corps humain et ses justifications dans l'antiquité," *Canadian Bulletin of Medical History* 10 (1993): 206.

85. *Peri archaiēs iatrikēs* 22 (L.1, 626–27) (Lloyd, *Hippocratic Medicine*, 84).

86. *Ibid.*

87. *Ibid.*

88. Galen, *Therapeutikēs methodou* 1.6 (K.10.47).

89. Galen, *Peri chreias tōn moriōn* 1.2 (K.2,2; trans. Margaret Tallmadge May, *Galen on the Usefulness of the Parts of the Body* [Ithaca, NY: Cornell University Press, 1968], vol. 1, 67–68).

90. Aristotle, *On the Soul* 415b.

91. Cited in François Delaporte, ed., *A Vital Rationalist: Selected Writings from Georges Canguilhem*, trans. Arthur Goldhammer (New York: Zone Books, 1994), 81. The ancient doctor Loxus, Elizabeth Evans relates, similarly explained in his treatise on physiognomy that "from the appearance of the body the quality of the soul may be changed, just as a breath infused into a pipe, or a flute or a trumpet is uniform, yet the pipe or the flute or the trumpet gives forth diverse sounds" (Elizabeth C. Evans, *Physiognomics in the Ancient World*, Transactions of the American Philosophical Society, new series vol. 59 [Philadelphia: American Philosophical Society, 1969], 11).

92. The sixth *fu* was the controversial *sanjiao* — the viscera "with a name but no form."

93. Sivin, *Traditional Medicine*, 120–21.

94. *Suwen* 11/37.

95. Ilza Veith, "Acupuncture Therapy — Past and Present," *Journal of the American Medical Association* 180 (1962): 478–79.

96. *Lingshu* 66/437.

97. In his extensive review of the European literature on ideas about the prolongation of life, Gerald Gruman concludes that "One of the most thought-provoking features of the evolution of prolongevitism is the striking contrast between China and the West." Whereas the emphasis on prolonging life was central to ancient and medieval China, in the West "the leading intellectual currents were extensively infiltrated with apologism, the belief that prolongevity is neither possible nor desirable." Gruman continues:

> That is not to say that prolongevitist tendencies were totally lacking in ancient Western civilization.... But in the West these tendencies remained fragmentary, while in China they were richly elaborated and made the subject of entire treatises. In the West, prolongevity was pushed to the periphery of the intellectual world or even driven underground, while in China it occupied a central position and attracted the attention of famous scholars, influential statesmen and, at times, the emperors themselves. (Gerald J. Gruman, *A History of Ideas about the Prolongation of Life: The Evolution of Prolongevity Hypotheses to 1800* [Philadelphia: American Philosophical Society, 1966], 28.)

98. Plato, *Epinomis* 976a–b (trans. Edith Hamilton and Huntington Cairns, eds., *The Collected Dialogues of Plato* [Princeton: Princeton University Press, 1973], 1519).

99. *Statesman* 299b.

100. Temkin, *Galenism*, 28–29.

101. On *pneuma* as an instrument of nature, see Aristotle, *Generation of Animals* 789b9f.

Chinese and Japanese

Names and Terms

Akatsuka Tadashi 赤塚忠
bafeng 八風
bafeng sishi 八風四時
bazheng 八政
benmo genye 本末根葉
bi 痺
Bi Gan 比干
Bian Que 扁鵲
bianse 變色
bianshi 砭石
biao 表
bigu 辟穀
bo 搏
boran bianse 勃然變色
boran zuose 勃然作色
bu buzu 補不足
buji 不及
buzhi chiman 不知持滿
bu zide 不自得
buzu 不足
Cai 蔡

Cao Xueqin 曹雪芹
Chabing zhinan 察病指南
Changsang Jun 長桑君
Chao Yuanfang 巢元方
chen 沈
chi (pond) 池
chi (qiemo inspection site; skin
   of the forearm) 尺
chu 出
Chu 楚
Chu Yong 儲泳
Chunyu Kun 淳于髡
Chunyu Yi 淳于意
Cihai 辭海
ciqi 辭氣
cong 從
Cui Zixu 崔紫虛
cun 寸
cunkou 寸口
da 達
dafeng 大風

331

dahui 大會

danzhong 膻中

dao 道

Daodejing 道德經

daoyin 導引

dashu 大數

de 德

Di 帝

dong 動

Dongguo Ya 東郭牙

dongmo 動脈

dou 道

Duan Yucai 段玉裁

duliang 度量

fangshu 房術

feng 風

feng hua ye 風化也

fengqi 風氣

fengshui 風水

fengsu 風俗

Fengsu tongyi 風俗通儀

fengtu 風土

fengzhan 風占

fenran zuose 忿然作色

fu (floating) 浮

fu (hollow viscera) 腑

fu feng zhe, qi ye 夫風者氣也

furan zuose 怫然作色

Gao Wu 高武

Gaozi 告子

gen 根

gong 工

gu 谷

guan (contemplate) 觀

guan (pulse position) 關

Guan Zhong 管仲

guanse yi kuixin
　　觀色以窺心

Guanzi 管子

Gujin tushu jicheng
　　古今圖書集成

guo 過

Guo Zhisui 郭志邃

Guofeng 國風

Guoyu 國語

hai 海

Han 漢

Han Fei 韓非

Hanfeizi 韓非子

Hanshu 漢書

haose 好色

he 合

He Xiu 何休

Hiraoka Teikichi 平岡負吉

hua (flower) 華

hua (slippery) 滑

Hua Shou 滑壽

Hua Tuo 華佗

Huainanzi 淮南子

Huan 桓

Huangdi neijing 黃帝內徑

huase 華色

hua se ye 華色也

Ji Zha 季札

Jiayijing 甲乙經
jifu 肌膚
jin 斤
Jin 晉
jing (conduit) 經
jing (quiet) 靜
jingluo 經絡
jingmo 經脈
Jingui yaolue 金匱要略
jingqi 精氣
Jingyue quanshu 景岳全書
jise 飢色
jiugong bafeng 九宮八風
jixiang 跡象
juan 卷
junzhu zhi guan 君主之官
Kato Munehiro 藤宗博
kong 空
Kong Fu 孔父
ku 枯
lai 來
laodong 勞動
Laozi 老子
li 理
li (inside) 裏
Li Gao 李呆
Li Shizhen 李時珍
Li Zhongzi 李中梓
liang 兩
liao 寮
Liezi 列子
liguan zhi shu 利關之術

Lingshu 靈樞
liu 流
liuli zhanshuan titiran
    流利展轉替替然
Lu 魯
Lülan 呂覽
Lunheng 論衡
Lunheng jiaoshi 論衡校釋
Lüshi chunqiu 呂氏春秋
Ma Jixing 馬繼興
man (repletion) 滿
mang 茫
mao 貌
Maruyama Masao 丸山昌郎
Mawangdui 馬王堆
mi 密
Mikami Yoshio 三上義夫
ming 明
mo 脈
Mojing 脈經
Mojue 脈訣
mokou 脈口
mo zhe, qixue zhi xian ye
    脈者氣血之先也
mu (longing) 慕
mu (to recruit) 募
Myakui bensei 脈位辯正
nan 難
nanfeng 南風
Nanjing 南風
nei 內
Neijing 內經

333

ni 逆

pimao 皮毛

Pinhu moxue 瀕湖脈學

qi 氣

Qi 齊

Qian Depei 錢德培

qiao 巧

qiaoyan lingse 巧顏伶色

qie 切

qiemo 切脈

Qin 秦

Qing 清

qingshen 輕身

qi rong se ye 其榮色也

qiu 丘

Qiwu lun 齊物論

qu 去

quan 泉

quchi 曲池

Quyi shuo 疑說

ru 入

Sanguo zhi 三國志

se (rough) 濇

se (color) 色

se boru ye 色勃如也

seli 色理

senan 色難

sesheng zhe 色盛者

seze 色澤

sezhe, qi zhi hua ye
　　色者，氣之華也

sha (disorders) 痧

shan 山

shang 上

Shang (dynasty) 商

shangfeng 傷風

shanggong 上工

Shanghanlun 傷寒論

Shazhang yuheng 痧張玉衡

shen 神

sheng (sagely) 聖

sheng 升

shengqi 生氣

shenming 神明

shi (fullness) 實

Shi Fa 施發

Shi Kuang 師曠

shifeng 實風

Shiji 史記

Shiming 釋名

shi se 失色

Shishu 十書

Shisi jing fahui 十四經發揮

Shujing 書經

Shuowen jiezi 說文解字

Sima Qian 司馬遷

Siyan juyao 四言舉要

Sizhen juewei 四珍訣微

Song 宋

Sun Muzi 孫穆子

sun youyu bu buzu
　　損有餘補不足

Sunzi 孫子

Suwen 素問

334

Taiping guangji 太平廣記
Taisu 太素
Taiyi 太一
Tang Zonghai 唐宗海
Tao Jiucheng 陶九成
tianqi (airs) 天氣
Tongshi 通史
wai 外
Waike jingyi 外科精義
wailian 外廉
Waitai miyao 外台秘要
wang (to gaze) 望
wang (to be absent) 亡
Wang Chong 王充
Wang Mang 王莽
Wang Shuhe 王叔和
Wang Tao 王
wangqi 望氣
wangse 望色
Wangsun Qing 王孫慶
wang yunwu 望雲物
wei (subtlety) 微
wei (wilts) 萎
weiqi 衛氣
wen (listen/smell) 聞
wen (question) 問
Wu 吳
wuchang 無常
wuse 五色
wuxing 五行
Xi (Duke) 僖
xi 谿

xia 下
xiagong 下工
Xiang (Duke) 襄
xie youyu 泄有餘
xiefeng 邪風
xieqi 邪氣
xin zhu mo 心主脈
xing (travel) 行
xing (shape) 形
xingse 形色
xingshen 形神
xingqi 形氣
xise 喜色
xizhong 郄中
xu (emptiness) 虛
Xu Shuwei 徐叔微
xuan 玄
xue (blood) 血
xuemo 血脈
xueqi 血氣
xufeng 虛風
Xunzi 荀子
xushi 虛實
xuwu 虛無
Yamada Keiji 山田慶兒
yan 顏
yang 陽
yangsheng 養生
yanqi 顏氣
yanse 顏色
yifeng yisu 易風易俗
Yi He 醫和

Yin (Duke) 隱

yin 陰

ying 盈

Yinyang shiyimo jiujing
　　陰陽十一脈灸經

Yizong bidu 醫宗必讀

youse 優色

youyu 有餘

yun chesan 雲撤散

zang (solid viscera) 臟

ze 澤

Zhai Yi 翟義

Zhang Liang 張良

Zhang Zhongjing 張仲景

Zhanguo ce 戰國策

Zhangjiashan 張家山

Zhao (Duke) 昭

Zheng 鄭

Zhenjia zhengyan 診家正言

Zhenjiu juying 鍼灸聚英

zhi yan 知言

zhong 中

zhongfeng 正風

zhonggong 中工

zhongri bu zi fan
　　終日不自反

Zhongzang jing 中藏經

Zhou 周

zhu (govern) 主

zhu (measure) 銖

Zhuangzi 莊子

Zhuning yuanhou lun
　　諸病源候論

Zhuogenglu 輟耕錄

zide 自得

Zi Gong 子貢

Zi Shen 梓慎

Zi Xia 子夏

zouli zhimi 奏理緻密

Zubi shiyimo jiujing
　　足臂十一脈灸經

zuose 作色

Zuozhuan 左傳

Index

ACKERKNECHT, ERWIN, 118–19, 120, 234.
Acupuncture, 43, 204–206, 220, 227, 228, 236.
Aegimius, 25–26, 28, 227n.20.
Aelianus, 131, 143.
Aelius Aristides, 68.
Aeschylus, 121, 245, 246.
Agathinus, 35.
Airs, Waters, Places, 137–38, 141–43, 204, 233–34, 235, 249, 269.
Akatsuka Tadashi, 236.
Akutagawa Ryūnosuke, 7–8.
Alberti, Leone Battista, 115–16.
Alexander, 33–34, 150.
Analects, 96–97, 103–104, 173–77 *passim*.
Anatomy, 30–32, 112–29, 159.
Anaxagoras, 125.
Archigenes, 35, 79.
Aretaeus, 207.
Aristotle, 88, 133, 202, 227, 229, 230; on articulation, 135–37, 147–48; on dissection, 30–31, 116, 122, 124, 157; on the heart, 151, 160; on Nature, 126–27, 147–48; on organism, 264; on *pneuma*, 261.
Aristoxenus, 33, 90–91, 291n.60.
Articulation, 134–43, 147.

Asclepiades, 230.
Atomists, 88.
Augustine, Saint, 262.
Avicenna, 81–85.

BACCHIUS, 32.
Baker, Thomas, 21.
Bian Que, 154, 162–63, 178.
Bible: Leviticus, 199.
Bichat, François, 213.
Blood: and food, 209, 216–18, 315n.64; and plethora, 208–17; and *pneuma*, 229–30; and *qi*, 229. *See also* Topological bleeding.
Bloodletting, 195–217; and acupuncture, 227, 228.
Bodde, Derk, 191.
Bodin, Jean, 250.
Body, 13–14, 271–72; governing principle of, 160–67; like plant, 186–91; in world, 262.
Bordeu, Théophile de, 66, 69, 80.
Boym, Michael, 21.
Brain, Peter, 197, 312n.44.
Burke, Richard, 67.

CANGUILHEM, GEORGES, 148–49.
Cao Xueqin, 191.
Celsus, 121, 197.
Chabing zhinan, 71, *84*, 99.

337

Chao Yuanfang, 251.
Chi, 52–54.
Chrysippus, 151.
Chunyu Yi, 70.
Cicero, 297n.55.
Clement of Alexandria, 216.
Color, in Chinese medicine, 167–91.
Confucius, 73–74, 96–97, 103–104,
  173–77 *passim*, 181–83 *passim*,
  200, 242, 244.

DAOISM, 73–74.
Demosthenes, 34, 150.
Diderot, Denis, 21, 61.
Diocles of Carystos, 116–17, 124.
Diodorus of Sicily, 136–37.
Diogenes, 160, 229, 261.
Dissection, 116–29; in China,
  155–60, 302nn.6, 7.
Donne, John, 17–18, 151.
Duan Yucai, 174.
Duncan, Daniel, 265.

EDELSTEIN, LUDWIG, 117.
Empiricist School, 33–34, 122.
"Emptiness," in Chinese medicine,
  218–28.
Encyclopédie, 21, 61.
Epler, D.C., 198.
Erasistratus, 117, 124, 211–12, 230,
  260.
Etang, Duchemin de l', 66.
Euripides, 135, 240, 246.
Exercise, 224–27.

FABRICA, 8, *11*, 123.
Floyer, John, 21–22, 37, 62–63, 64,
  99.
Forke, Alfred, 50.
Formey, Johan L., 37.
Fouquet, Henri, 65–66.
Friedlander, Paul, 126.
"Fullness," in Chinese medicine,
  218–28.

GALEN, 12, 76, 185, 189, 224, 227,
  228, 260–61, 263–64; on
  anatomy, 122–24, 127–28, 161,
  162; on bloodletting, 195, 197,
  200, 201, 206–15 *passim*; on muscles, 130–31, 133, 143–51 *passim*,
  161; on pulse, 20, 23, 25–29,
  34–36, 67–68, 76, 78–80, 85, 90,
  95, 230, 231, 286n.16, 287n.17.
Gao Wu, 198.
Gaozi, 176.
Gruman, Gerald, 329n.97.
Guofeng, 243–44.

HACKFORTH, R., 87–89.
Hafenreffer, Samuel, 81, *82*.
Hall, Marshall, 196.
Harris, C.R.S., 68.
Harvey, William, 196, 311n.22.
Heberden, William, 69, 77, 80.
Heister, Lorenz, 196.
Heraclides of Erythrae, 32–33.
Hercules, 135, 139, *140*.
Hercules Saxonia, 20.
Herodotus, 88, 129, 141, 241.
Herophilus, 28, 30, 31–32, 35, 36,
  79, 85–86, 90, 117, 150–51, 260.
He Xiu, 239.
Hippocrates of Cos, 23.
Hippocratic corpus, 23, 28–29, 118,
  129, 262–63; *Airs, Waters, Places*,
  137–39, 141–43, 204, 233–34,
  235, 249; on blood, 196–97, 200;
  on the heart, 124, 149; *On the
  Seed*, 135; on topological bleed-
  ing, 201, 202–204, 206–10 *passim*,
  213; on winds, 246–50.
Hiraoka Teikichi, 236.
Homer, 146, 241, 245, 249.
Horses, blood vessels of, 41, 282n.75.
Hua Shou, 8, 10, 107.
Hua Tuo, 102–103, 184, 224,
  292n.75, 304n.37.
Huangdi neijing, see Neijing.

JAEGER, WERNER, 89.
Joints, *see* Articulation.
Jombert, Charles-Antoine, 112, 115.
Jones, Peter Murray, 205.

KATŌ MUNEHIRO, 40.
Kircher, Athanasius, 81, *83*.

LAOZI, 73, 220.
Leonardo da Vinci, 115, 292n.4.
Li Gao, 47, 98, 198.
Lippman, Edward, 86–88.
Li Shizhen, 98.
Littré, Emile, 197.
Li Zhongzi, 47, 72–73, 98.
Lu Gwei-djen, 44.
Lu Shouyan, 43–44.
Lycus, 131, 143.

MAGNUS, 79.
Ma Jixing, 43.
Marinus, 143, 146.
Marquet, François Nicolas, 81, *83*,
    289n.45.
Mawangdui manuscripts, 41–44, 217.
Melampus, 30.
Mencius, 104, 171–76 *passim*, 180,
    181, 190, 191.
Menstruation, 227, 318n.112.
Menuret de Chambaud, J.J., 61–62,
    289n.45.
Mikami Yoshio, 155–56.
Ming, Emperor, 179.
Mnesitheus, 135.
Mo, 44, 48–51, 100–102; as circular,
    160. *See also Qiemo.*
Mojing, 40, 65, 72, 93–96.
Mojue, 21, 22, *100*.
Montesquieu, Baron de, 251.
Mueller, Johannes, 213.
Muscles, history of, 112–16, 129–51.
Music: and pulse, 81–91; and wind:
    242–45.
Myron, 91, *92*.

NANJING, 12, 40, 45–46, 153.
Needham, Joseph, 44.
Neijing, 12, 38, 41, 252–54, 280n.65.
Nihell, James, 66.
North, Milo, 66–67.
Nutton, Vivian, 68.

ODYSSEY, THE, 241.
On the Movement of Muscles, 144–45.
On the Usefulness of the Parts, 123.
Organs, concept of, 263–66.
Origen, 262.
Ozanam, Charles, 22, 51.

PADEL, RUTH, 245–46.
Palmomantics, 30.
Parthenon metopes, *113*, 129.
Parts of Animals, 127, 157.
Peck, A.L., 128.
Pelops, 131, 143.
Peterson, Eugen, 88.
Philebus, 86–88.
Physiognomics, 134, 142.
Pindar, 121.
Plants, as metaphors for body,
    186–91.
Plato, 119, 121, 129; on athletics,
    139; on the brain, 160; on medi-
    cine, 268–69; *Philebus*, 86–88; on
    the soul, 216–17; *Timaeus*, 125–26,
    230; on wind, 235.
Plethora, *see* Blood.
Polemo, 185.
Pollaiuolo, Antonio, 112, *114*.
Pollitt, J.J., 88–89.
Porkert, Manfred, 267.
Praxagoras of Cos, 28, 29–30, 31–32.
Pulse, 18–37, *56, 57, 58, 59*, 65–67,
    69–70, 75–91, 150–51, 230–31.

QI, 102–104, 223
Qian Depei, 38.
Qiemo, 22, *26–27*, 37–55, 70–75,
    93–104, 287n.22.

Rhythmos, 88–91.
Rivière, Lazarus, 250.
Rucco, Julius, 20.
Rufus of Ephesus, 25–26, 28, 30, 31, 122, 146.
Rush, Benjamin, 20.
Ruskin, John, 189.

Satyrus, 68.
Scythians, 137–38, 204–205.
Se, 172–85. *See also* Color.
Sexual intercourse, 228.
Shi, see "Fullness."
Shi Fa, 71, 81, *84*, 99.
Shisijing fahui, 8, *10*.
Sigerist, Henry, 120, 234.
Sima Qian, 164, 169, 239.
Sivin, Nathan, 265.
Snell, Bruno, 120, 300n.102.
Sophocles, 135.
Steno, Nicholas, 301n.110.
Strabo, 136.
Struthius, Josephus, 68, 81, *82*.
Synopsis on Pulses, 25.

Tang Zonghai, 37.
Theophrastus, 124.
Timaeus, 125–26, 230.
Topological bleeding, 201–207, 313n.49.

Valéry, Paul, 13–14.
Veith, Ilza, 266.
Verbeke, Gérard, 260.
Vernant, Jean–Pierre, 146.
Vesalius, 8, *11*, 123.

Wang Chong, 50, 178, 236, 239.
Wang Shuhe, 40, 49–50, 93–96, 98.
Wangsun Qing, dissection of, 155–59.
Waterton, Charles, 196.
Winds, 164–65, 221–22, 233–42, 268–70; and music, 242–45; in Greek medicine, 246–51, 259–65;

in Chinese medicine, 251–59, 265–68.
Wotton, William, 21.

Xenophon, 125.
Xu, see "Emptiness."

Yamada Keiji, 44, 197.
Yi He, 252.
Yinyang shiyimo jiujing, 41–44.

Zhangjiashan Tombs, 48, 282n.76.
Zhang Liang, 217.
Zhao Da, 254.
Zhuangzi, 73, 174, 176, 184, 223, 244–45.
Zubi shiyimo jiujing, 41–44.